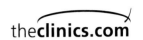

CLINICS IN SPORTS MEDICINE

Infectious Disease and Sports Medicine

GUEST EDITORS
James R. Borchers, MD
Thomas M. Best, MD, PhD, FACSM

CONSULTING EDITOR
Mark D. Miller, MD

July 2007 • Volume 26 • Number 3

SAUNDERS

An Imprint of Elsevier, Inc.
PHILADELPHIA   LONDON   TORONTO   MONTREAL   SYDNEY   TOKYO

W.B. SAUNDERS COMPANY
A Division of Elsevier Inc.

1600 John F. Kennedy Blvd. • Suite 1800 • Philadelphia, Pennsylvania 19103

http://www.theclinics.com

CLINICS IN SPORTS MEDICINE   Volume 26, Number 3
July 2007   ISSN 0278-5919
Editor: Debora Dellapena   ISBN-13: 978-1-4160-5056-8
                                                   ISBN-10: 1-4160-5056-6

Clinics in Sports Medicine (ISSN 0278-5919) is published quarterly by Elsevier Inc., 360 Park Avenue South, New York, NY 10010-1710. Months of publication are January, April, July, and October. Business and Editorial Offices: 1600 John F. Kennedy Blvd., Suite 1800, Philadelphia, PA 19103-2899. Customer Service Offices: 6277 Sea Harbor Drive, Orlando, FL 32887-4800. Periodicals postage paid at New York, NY, and additional mailing offices. Subscription prices are $205.00 per year (US individuals), $313.00 per year (US institutions), $103.00 per year (US students), $232.00 per year (Canadian individuals), $371.00 per year (Canadian institutions), $135.00 (Canadian students), $265.00 per year (foreign individuals), $371.00 per year (foreign institutions), and $135.00 per year (foreign students). Foreign air speed delivery is included in all *Clinics* subscription prices. All prices are subject to change without notice. POSTMASTER: Send address changes to *Clinics in Sports Medicine*, Elsevier Periodicals Customer Service, 6277 Sea Harbor Drive, Orlando, FL 32887-4800. **Customer Service: 1-800-654-2452 (US). From outside of the US, call 1-407-345-4000.** E-mail: hhspcs@harcourt.com.

Clinics in Sports Medicine is covered in *Index Medicus, Current Contents/Clinical Medicine, Excerpta Medica,* and *ISI/Biomed.*

Printed in the United States of America.

ELSEVIER
SAUNDERS

CLINICS IN SPORTS MEDICINE

Infectious Disease and Sports Medicine

CONSULTING EDITOR

MARK D. MILLER, MD, Professor, Department of Orthopaedic Surgery; Head, Division of Sports Medicine, University of Virginia Health System, Charlottesville, Virginia

GUEST EDITORS

JAMES R. BORCHERS, MD, Assistant Clinical Professor of Family Medicine, Division of Sports Medicine, The Ohio State University Sports Medicine Center, Team Physician, Department of Athletics, The Ohio State University, Columbus, Ohio

THOMAS M. BEST, MD, PhD, FACSM, Professor and Pomerene Chair, Family Medicine; Chief, Division of Sports Medicine; Director, Primary Care Sports Medicine Fellowship, The Ohio State University, Columbus, Ohio

CONTRIBUTORS

JAMES R. BORCHERS, MD, Assistant Clinical Professor of Family Medicine, Division of Sports Medicine, The Ohio State University Sports Medicine Center; Team Physician, Department of Athletics, The Ohio State University, Columbus, Ohio

P. GUNNAR BROLINSON, DO, FAOASM, FAAFP, Chief of Sports Medicine, Virginia College of Osteopathic Medicine; Head Team Physician, Virginia Tech Sports Medicine, Blacksburg, Virginia

CATHY L. CANTOR, MD, MBA, Associate Director, Sports Care/Sports Medicine Fellowship, The Toledo Hospital, Promedica Health System; Director of Women's Sports, University of Toledo, Toledo, Ohio

KELLEY L. CLEM, MD, MS, Ohio Orthopedic Center of Excellence, Upper Arlington, Ohio

WILLIAM W. DEXTER, MD, FACSM, Director, Sports Medicine Program; Assistant Director, Family Practice Residency Program, Maine Medical Center, Portland, Maine

PIERRE D'HEMECOURT, MD, Director, Primary Care Sports Medicine, Harvard University, Children's Hospital of Boston, Boston, Massachusetts

JASON J. DIEHL, MD, Assistant Professor of Clinical Family Medicine, Division of Sports Medicine, Department of Family Medicine, The Ohio State University Sports Medicine Center, Columbus, Ohio

DAN ELLIOTT, DO, Fellow, Primary Care Sports Medicine, Virginia Center for Athletic Medicine, Christopher Newport University; Head Team Physician, Newport News, Virginia

MATTHEW R. GAMMONS, MD, Assistant Clinical Professor, Department of Family and Community Medicine, Medical College of Wisconsin, Milwaukee, Wisconsin; Killington Medical Clinic, Vermont Orthopedic Clinic, Killington, Vermont

LAURA M. GOTTSCHLICH, DO, Assistant Professor, Department of Family and Community Medicine, Medical College of Wisconsin, Milwaukee, Wisconsin

ROBERT G. HOSEY, MD, Associate Professor, Departments of Family and Community Medicine and Orthopaedics; Director, Primary Care Sports Medicine Fellowship, University of Kentucky Chandler Medical Center, Lexington, Kentucky

STEVEN J. KARAGEANES, DO, FAOASM, Director, Sports Medicine Fellowship; Associate Director, Family Practice Residency, Oakwood Healthcare System; Clinical Associated Professor, Michigan State University College of Osteopathic Medicine; Head Team Physician, Wayne State University, Plymouth, Michigan

JOEL M. KARY, MD, Fellow, South Bend Sports Medicine Fellowship, Memorial Sports Medicine Institute, South Bend, Indiana

ROGER J. KRUSE, MD, FACSM, Director, Sports Care/Sports Medicine Fellowship, The Toledo Hospital, Promedica Health System; Head Physician, University of Toledo, Toledo, Ohio

MARK LAVALLEE, MD, CSCS, FACSM, Co-Director, South Bend Sports Medicine Fellowship; Director, Memorial Sports Medicine Institute, South Bend, Indiana; Team Physician, Vice Chair, Sports Medicine Committee, USA Weightlifting, US Olympic Training Center, Colorado Springs, Colorado; Medical Director, International Weightlifting Federation–Masters Program, Budapest, Hungary

DONALD C. LEMAY, DO, Assistant Professor, Department of Family Medicine, The Ohio State University; Team Physician, Athletics, The Ohio State University Division of Sports Medicine, The Ohio State University Sports Medicine Center, Columbus, Ohio

ANTHONY LUKE, MD, MPH, Assistant Professor, Departments of Orthopaedic Surgery and Family and Community Medicine; Director, Primary Care Sports Medicine, University of California San Francisco, San Francisco, California

MARK W. NIEDFELDT, MD, Associate Professor, Departments of Orthopaedic Surgery, Family and Community Medicine, and Cell Biology, Neurobiology, and Anatomy, Medical College of Wisconsin, Milwaukee, Wisconsin

CONTRIBUTORS continued

CLIFTON L. PAGE, MD, Primary Care Sports Medicine Fellow, Division of Sports Medicine, Department of Family Medicine, The Ohio State University Sports Medicine Center, Columbus, Ohio

CHARLES S. PETERSON, MD, Instructor of Family Medicine, Mayo Clinic College of Medicine, Arizona Sports Medicine Center, Scottsdale, Arizona

JASON J. PIROZZOLO, DO, CentraCare Hospital, Orlando, Florida

MICHAEL D. PLEACHER, MD, McKay-Dee Sports Medicine, Ogden, Utah

RICHARD E. RODENBERG, MD, Program Director, Sports Medicine Fellowship, Grant Medical Center, Columbus, Ohio

PETER E. SEDGWICK, MD, Fellow, Sports Medicine Fellowship Program, Sports Medicine Program, Maine Medical Center, Portland, Maine

CHRISTINA T. SMITH, MD, OAA Orthopaedic Specialists, Sports Medicine Institute, Allentown, Pennsylvania

CRAIG C. YOUNG, MD, Medical Director of Sports Medicine, Professor, Departments of Orthopaedic Surgery and Family and Community Medicine, Medical College of Wisconsin, Milwaukee, Wisconsin

CLINICS IN SPORTS MEDICINE

Infectious Disease and Sports Medicine

CONTENTS   VOLUME 26 • NUMBER 3 • JULY 2007

> Exercise has a variable effect on the immune system. The underlying reasons for this variability are multifactorial and include infectious, neuroedocrine, and metabolic factors, with nutritional status of the athlete and the training load playing a role. Environmental factors such as living quarters, travel requirements, and the type of sport (team versus individual) also contribute to infectious risk. Regarding the direct effect of exercise on the immune system, moderate exercise seems to exert a protective effect, whereas repeated bouts of strenuous exercise can result in immune dysfunction. Understanding the relationship between exercise and infectious disease has important potential implications for public health and for clinicians caring for athletes and athletic teams.

> The sports medicine physician may face challenging issues regarding infectious diseases when dealing with teams or highly competitive athletes who have difficulties taking time off to recover. One must treat the individual sick athlete and take the necessary precautions to contain the spread of communicable disease to the surrounding team, staff, relatives, and other contacts. This article reviews preventive strategies for infectious disease in athletes, including immunization recommendations and prophylaxis guidelines, improvements in personal hygiene and prevention of spread of infectious organisms by direct contact, insect-borne disease precautions, and prevention of sexually transmitted diseases. A special emphasis on immunizations focuses on pertussis, influenza, and meningococcal prophylaxis.

> Upper respiratory tract infections (URTIs) represent the most common acute illnesses in the general population and account for the leading acute diagnoses in the outpatient setting. Given the athlete's expectation to

return to activity as soon as possible, the sports medicine physician should be able to accurately diagnose and aggressively treat these illnesses. This article discusses the common pathogens, diagnosis, treatment options, and return-to-play decisions for URTIs, with a focus on the common cold, sinusitis, pharyngitis, and infectious mononucleosis in the athlete.

Pulmonary and cardiac infections in the athlete can have a wide range of presentations and complications. These infections may present few problems for the training athlete or become life threatening. The team physician must be able to make an accurate diagnosis, give the appropriate treatment, understand the potential complications, and ensure proper follow-up and return-to-play protocols.

Bacterial skin dermatoses are common in athletes, and it is the role of team physicians to be able to recognize and treat such problems. Despite the skin's role as an efficient barrier, a moist environment coupled with frequent skin trauma and contact by athletes with equipment and other players predispose to acquiring infections. In the past 10 years, there has been a dramatic rise in methicillin-resistant *Staphylococcus aureus* (MRSA) infections. This article discusses community-acquired MRSA infections among athletes and focuses on the recognition of, management of, and return-to-play guidelines for common bacterial skin infections in athletes. Some of the more unusual bacterial infections that may present in this population are also reviewed.

Fungal and viral cutaneous infections are common among athletes and can develop quickly into widespread outbreaks. To prevent such outbreaks, the team physician must be familiar with common cutaneous infections including tinea corporis, tinea capitis, tinea pedis, herpes simplex, molluscum contagiosum, and human papillomaviruses. Appropriate treatment and management of these infections allows the athlete to safely return to play and safeguards teammates and opponents against the spread of these diseases.

HIV/AIDS is considered a worldwide pandemic, with continued increases in the number of newly diagnosed cases and persons living long-term with the disease. Athletes may be at risk of infection based on behaviors associated with participation in their sport and away from competition. The sports medicine physician must be aware of the risk of HIV/AIDS in the athlete, diagnosis and treatment options, the effect of HIV/AIDS on exercise, and strategies for prevention of HIV/AIDS in athletic competition.

Blood-borne infections are transmitted by way of direct blood contact from one individual to another from injured skin or a mucous membrane. Blood-borne infections can also be transmitted through blood doping and drug abuse and through sexual contact. Risk factors for hepatitis B virus (HBV) HBV infection include travel to regions with endemic hepatitis. Prevention of blood-borne pathogens in the student-athlete should focus on traditional transmission routes and off-the-field behavior because experts believe that field transmission of blood-borne pathogens is minimal. Worldwide, HBV, hepatitis C virus (HCV), and HIV are the most common pathogens encountered. This article focuses on HBV and HCV as being the most prevalent in athletics.

Gastrointestinal (GI) infections can be troublesome and debilitating to athletes and difficult to manage for sports medicine physicians. A clinician should obtain a comprehensive medical history of the athlete whenever symptoms of the GI tract appear. The predominant chief complaint in GI infections is diarrhea. Athletes may need a comprehensive physical examination to appropriately diagnose the ailment and to determine the need for more aggressive treatment. Multiple laboratory tests exist to aid in diagnosing the infectious pathogen causing gastroenteritis. This article discusses GI infections caused by viral, parasitic, bacterial, and food-borne infectious pathogens. The epidemiology, pathogenesis, history, symptoms, mode of transmission, laboratory detection, treatment, and prevention of these infections are reviewed.

Collegiate athletes are common reservoirs for infectious disease agents. Specific training regimens, living arrangements, and high-risk behaviors may influence the athlete's risk of contracting a variety of infectious diseases. The sports medicine physician plays an important role in recognizing, appropriately treating, designing prevention strategies for, and making return-to-activity decisions for athletes who have infectious diseases.

CLINICS IN SPORTS MEDICINE

Clin Sports Med 26 (2007) xiii

CLINICS IN SPORTS MEDICINE

Foreword

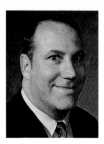

Mark D. Miller, MD
Consulting Editor

A s a "bone doctor" I am always in search of topics of interest to other sports medicine clinicians. My interest, and the interests of my colleagues in orthopedic sports medicine, also has been broadened recently with the advent of the Subspecialty Certification in Sports Medicine examination that will be offered for the first time this November. This is stuff we all have to know!

Therefore, it is my distinct pleasure to introduce this issue of the *Clinics in Sports Medicine* that focuses on infectious disease in sports medicine. With the recent training room scare involving multidrug-resistant *Staphylococcus aureus*, this topic is indeed timely. I invited Dr. Tom Best, who has already helped us prepare for our upcoming examination by putting together a great lecture on medical topics for our Instructional Course Lecture at last winter's annual meeting of the American Academy of Orthopaedic Surgeons, to spearhead this issue. He enlisted the assistance of his colleague, Dr. James Borchers, to put together a truly phenomenal issue. As you can see from the Table of Contents, this issue covers all aspects of infectious disease in sports—from all organ systems and all types of infections. Indeed, infection, unlike beauty, is not only skin deep!

Mark D. Miller, MD
Professor, Department of Orthopedic Surgery
Head, Division of Sports Medicine
University of Virginia Health System
P.O. Box 800753
Charlottesville, VA 22903-0753, USA

E-mail address: mdm3p@virginia.edu

0278-5919/07/$ – see front matter
doi:10.1016/j.csm.2007.04.013

Clin Sports Med 26 (2007) xv–xvi

CLINICS IN SPORTS MEDICINE

Preface

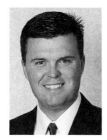
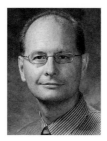

James R. Borchers, MD
Thomas M. Best, MD, PhD, FACSM

Guest Editors

The study of infectious disease and sports medicine seem to have very little in common, but in fact the overlap between the two fields is more significant than one initially might think. Often an active individual is confronted with the scenario of participating in an athletic event or activity while facing an infectious disease. It is imperative that the sports medicine practitioner understand the interaction that exists between the athlete, the athlete's activity, and a diagnosis of infectious disease.

This issue of the *Clinics in Sports Medicine* highlights some of the most common issues in infectious disease facing the Sports Medicine practitioner caring for athletes. The opening article explores the effects of exercise on the immune system to provide the reader with basic knowledge about the impact of exercise on various aspects of the immune response. Prevention of infectious disease is paramount for the care of the athlete, and the second article explores important strategies. The following articles offer the reader an opportunity to review the care of the athlete who has various infectious disease processes, from upper respiratory and gastrointestinal infectious disease to more complex issues including cardiopulmonary and blood-borne pathogens. Two articles are devoted to infectious disease of the skin, and one article discusses specific care of the athlete who has HIV. Finally, three articles are dedicated to infectious disease in specific populations: the collegiate athlete, the "extreme sport" athlete, and the athlete competing at the international elite level.

Evidence-based medicine is one of the strongest tools any practitioner has for appropriate practice in medicine today. Statistics, probabilities, likelihoods, and ratios are at the core of evidence-based medicine. Defining the evidence-based practice of medicine is an evolving process that requires sound research and

0278-5919/07/$ – see front matter
doi:10.1016/j.csm.2007.04.014
sportsmed.theclinics.com

analysis to guide the practitioner in clinical decision making. Many areas of sports medicine are lacking in good evidence-based practice guidelines and rely only on expert opinion for the basis of practice. The authors of this issue are to be commended for attempting to present the best evidence-based practices and guidelines in their review of the various infectious disease topics. It is imperative that the practitioner remain vigilant for new infectious disease processes and their effect on an athletic/active population.

We extend our thanks to Mark Miller, MD, for the opportunity to present this edition of the *Clinics in Sports Medicine*. Special thanks go to the staff at Elsevier and especially to Deb Dellapena for assistance in preparing this collection of articles. We also thank the authors for their time and effort in preparing these articles.

James R. Borchers, MD
The Ohio State University Sports Medicine Center, 3rd Floor
The Ohio State University
2050 Kenny Road
Columbus, OH 43221, USA

E-mail address: james.borchers@osumc.edu

Thomas M. Best, MD, PhD, FACSM
The Ohio State University
2050 Kenny Road
Columbus, OH 43221, USA

E-mail address: tom.best@osumc.edu

Exercise and the Immune System

P. Gunnar Brolinson, DO, FAOASM, FAAFP[a,*],
Dan Elliott, DO[b]

[a]Virginia College of Osteopathic Medicine, Virginia Tech Sports Medicine,
112 Merryman Center, Blacksburg, VA 24061, USA
[b]Primary Care Sports Medicine, Virginia Center for Athletic Medicine,
Christopher Newport University, Newport News, VA 23606, USA

One of the most common reasons for poor performance at a major sporting event is an acute respiratory infection. A common perception among elite athletes and coaches is that heavy exercise may lower resistance and is a predisposing factor for upper respiratory tract infections (URTI) [1]. Many elite athletes have reported significant bouts with respiratory infections that have interfered with their ability to compete and train [1]. In juxtaposition to this concept is the common belief among many individuals that regular exercise is beneficial to the immune system and may confer some resistance to infection [1]. A 1989 *Runner's World* subscriber survey revealed that 61% of 700 runners reported fewer colds since beginning to run, whereas only 4% experienced more colds [2]. The National Center for Health Statistics reported that acute respiratory conditions (primarily the common cold and influenza) have an annual incidence rate of 90 per 100 persons, imposing substantial morbidity and economic burden on families [3]. The Centers for Disease Control and Prevention estimates there are 425 million colds and episodes of flu annually in the United States, with medical care and lost work costs estimated at $2.5 billion annually [4]. Therefore, understanding the relationship between exercise and infectious disease has important potential implications for public health and for clinicians caring for athletes and athletic teams. What are the implications for practicing clinicians? Does exercise predispose to, or protect from, infectious disease? What are the effects of exercise on infectious disease? How does infection affect athletic performance? Are there guidelines for exercise during acute or chronic infections? Is there an immune link between exercise and cancer? What about exercise, aging, and immunity? Are there gender-specific issues regarding exercise and immunity? Is there a role for nutritional supplements? What is the role of drug (antibiotic) therapy?

*Corresponding author. E-mail address: techdo@vt.edu (P.G. Brolinson).

0278-5919/07/$ – see front matter
doi:10.1016/j.csm.2007.04.011

THE IMMUNE SYSTEM

The immune system is very complex and essential for maintaining health. Dysfunction can lead to a wide variety of diseases. The immune system comprises two basic components: the innate immune system and the adaptive immune system. Elements of the innate system include exterior defenses (such as the skin and mucous membranes), nonspecific phagocytic leukocytes, and serum proteins [4]. Pathogens that escape these initial outer barriers then come in contact with the adaptive system, which is made up of T and B cells. When this system is activated, cells with the ability to recognize specific microbes are generated. Unlike the innate system, the adaptive system develops gradually but exhibits memory and reacts quicker with subsequent exposure, which in turn results in a more comprehensive and efficient adaptive defense mechanisms with each repeated exposure to that specific pathogen. Together, these two elements provide a formidable obstacle to the establishment and long-term survival of infectious agents [5].

THE INNATE SYSTEM

The largest organ in the body, the skin, provides the initial blockade to infection. Many natural openings to body cavities and glands, however, provide entry for infectious agents. Protection at these sites is provided in the form of mucus, enzymes, and secretory immunoglobulins. Certain organs such as the lung and stomach also prevent entrance into the bloodstream. Characteristics specific for these organs, such as alveolar macrophages and low pH, respectively, provide protection from further invasion [5]. When these lines of defense are penetrated, the invading organism faces further compromise by the nonspecific fixed monocyte-macrophage system that lines the sinusoids and vasculature of organs such as the liver, spleen, and bone marrow. After a foreign substance enters the body, the inflammatory response begins generating an intricate cascade of events. Initially, circulating proteins and blood cells interact with the invading organism, initiating increased blood flow to the affected tissue. This, vasodilation in turn, results in the four classic signs of inflammation: rubor (redness), calor (heat), tumor (edema), and dolor (pain) [6]. This reaction essentially enhances the delivery of the immune system elements necessary to propagate the inflammatory response on a more microscopic level. These inflammatory mediators perpetuate the increased blood flow and result in increased capillary permeability, allowing diffusion of larger molecules across the endothelium. These molecules often play a role in eliminating the pathogen or in further enhancing the inflammatory response [5]. Such elements include the complement system, chemotactic factors, polymorphonuclear leukocytes, phagocytes, and components of the adaptive system such as immunospecific antibodies. Actual cell death then occurs with the extracellular release of inflammatory mediators such as free radicals and granular enzymes. Lysis of bacterial, viral, and cancer cells is also accomplished by natural killer cells. These large granular lymphocytes also prevent growth and establishment of foreign pathogens. It must remembered that these systems are described separately, but in vivo, these systems are intricately interwoven and only function appropriately when linked with the other system [5,7].

THE ADAPTIVE SYSTEM

The adaptive system provides its skill of fending off invaders by three unique methods. The first is the ability to recognize antigenic markers on specific pathogens. The second is the ability to supply a cellular and molecular assault on the invading organisms. The final aspect of this destructive triad is the capability of recalling previous invaders, which in turn accelerates and potentiates subsequent responses to the same agent or antigen. The cells that compose the adaptive system are antibodies, T cells, and B cells. Respectively, these cells are responsible for the recognition, effector, and memory functions of the adaptive system [7]. For this complex cascade to occur, an initial activation must occur, termed clonal selection. After a specific antigen has been recognized by a B cell's receptor, a progeny of B and T lymphocytes (specific for the inducing antigen) are created. These daughter B cells may proliferate into plasma cells capable of generating antibodies or into memory cells that function as the recognizing sentinel cell. As the number of these specific cells increases, so does the ability to react and respond to a future invasion, providing resistance to clinical disease [5]. This memory response is the fundamental basis for the use of vaccinations against certain diseases such as influenza, polio, varicella, measles, meningitis, and so forth. When the body is exposed to one of these pathogens, two possible responses may occur: cellular or humoral. As mentioned earlier, the T cells and B cells, respectively, carry out these responses. Cellular immunity is accomplished by a variety of T cells [6]. These cells do not secrete antibodies but create certain types of cells programmed with specific responsibilities. The helper T cell suppresses or activates certain immunologic mechanisms of other cells, whereas the cytotoxic T cell directly lyses pathogens, resulting in cell death. The activated T cell also provides the ability to secrete cytotoxic or immunomodulating cytokines such as tumor necrosis factor and interleukin 2 [5,7]. In contrast to the rapid onset of biologic response seen with the B-cell line, the T-cell activation is usually not recognized until 24 to 48 hours after the initial antigen challenge. An example of this reaction is the delayed-type hypersensivity, such as the tuberculin purified protein derivative test. T cell–mediated immune response is also responsible for the rejection of transplant tissue grafts and the suppression of neoplastic cells. Deficiency of the T-cell progeny can lead to serious life-threatening disease such as seen in patients who have AIDS [6]. The humoral response is dictated by the versatile B cell that can proliferate into plasma cells or memory cells, as described earlier. Plasma cells have the ability to create antigenic-specific antibodies. The antibodies, or immunoglobulins, can be found in a variety of body fluids conveying external (saliva) and internal (serum) protection. There are different classes of immunoglobulins based on the molecular structure, size, and function. Immunoglobulin (Ig)G is the most prevalent antibody in serum and is responsible for induced immunity against bacteria and other microorganisms. IgA is considered a secretory immunoglobulin due its protein being synthesized in the epithelium, allowing its secretion into the saliva, tears, colostrum, and mucus. This allows it to be secreted into the saliva, tears, colostrum, and mucus. IgM is unique, in that is the first immunoglobulin to be released after the initial antigenic challenge, thus providing resistance early in the course of an infection. Finally, IgE is an important player in the allergic response because it preferentially binds cells that store and release mediators of allergy and anaphylaxis, such as mast cells and basophils. The allergic response varies, from hives, rhinitis, and asthma to severe and sometimes fatal anaphylaxis. In contrast to the delayed response of the T cell, the antibodies can induce an immediate immunologic response known as an immediate hypersensitivity reaction. A specific example of this reaction is an anaphylactic reaction in which an antibody that is fixed to a mast cell binds to its specific antigen, generating an acute inflammatory reaction [5]. The mast cell degranulates, releasing certain mediators of the allergic response, including histamine (a potent vasodilator) and leukotrienes (smooth muscle contractors). Immune complexes that activate the plasma complement system cause other immediate reactions. The complement system comprises numerous distinct circulating proteins that, when activated, result in edema, chemotaxis (influx of activated phagotic cells), and local inflammatory changes [7]. Overall, the combination and the intricate interaction between the innate and adaptive immune systems provide an extensive system to prevent and destroy pathogenic organisms.

SPORTS IMMUNOLOGY

Sports immunology is a relatively new field that examines the interaction of physical, psychologic, and environmental stress on immune function. Over the last 100 years, there have been more than 600 articles published in this area. Most (>60%) have been published since 1990. As late as 1984, some investigators believed that "there is no clear experimental or clinical evidence that exercise will alter the frequency or severity of human infections" [4]. More recently, clinicians and scientists have begun to understand the complex interaction between exercise and immune function. For the purposes of this review, the authors define *exercise* as the leisure-time application of physical activity. *Training* is the result of repetitive bouts of exercise, and *fitness* is the result of consistent training.

IMPACT OF EXERCISE ON THE IMMUNE SYSTEM

A large bank of scientific, clinical, and epidemiologic data supports the concept of positive and negative impacts of exercise on the immune system, including the American College of Sports Medicine position papers and the Surgeon General's report on physical activity and health. These effects are highly variable, depending on the nature and intensity of exercise. Currently, the authors define vigorous exercise as 5 to 60 minutes at 70% to 80% aerobic capacity and moderate exercise as 5 to 60 minutes at 40% to 60% aerobic capacity.

THE CELLULAR EFFECTS OF EXERCISE

The specific cause for the difference in URTI incidence has been demonstrated on a microscopic level. Cellular response to physical activity is seen with natural killer cell activity, neutrophil function, and lymphocytic response. Several studies have reproduced this concept; however, few have related the actual cellular response to the presence of clinical disease. There has been a great deal of research into the effects of exercise on secretory immunoglobulins, specifically IgA. As described earlier, IgA is the predominant antibody contained in secretions of the mucosal immune system and, therefore, one of the body's first lines of defense against invading upper respiratory pathogens. Since the late 1970s, researchers have demonstrated a disappearance of immunoglobulins in athletes [1,8]. Mackinnon and colleagues [9] reported an inverse relationship in URTI and secretory IgA presence. This finding has led to further investigation not only in the concentration of IgA but also in the rate of mucosal IgA secretion. Recent research has been more clinically relevant, searching for a direct relationship between cellular change and disease. A longitudinal study by Fahlman and Engels [10] reported that one year of American football resulted in a significant decrease in secretory IgA and the secretion rate of IgA. These investigators also related these findings to an increase in URTI. This drop in IgA effectiveness has also been shown to occur with only 1 hour of intensive activity. Novas and colleagues [11] also demonstrated that secretion rate and IgA concentration were directly associated with the amount of training during the previous day and week. It must be noted that these previous studies examined intensive activity. Other recent studies have investigated the effects of moderate exercise on IgA production, with the hypothesis that moderate activity would improve the body's immune function. Klentrou and colleagues [12] used an aerobic exercise program comprising three 30-minute sessions per week at 75% maximal heart rate. Salivary IgA concentration and secretion rates at rest were significantly increased in the group undergoing regular, moderate exercise. It appears that the level of intensity is the important factor in affecting the concentration and the secretory rate of IgA, which is a primary deterrent of clinical URTI. Another important player of innate immunology is the natural killer cell. Most studies reveal enhanced natural killer cell activity in athletes versus nonathletes [13]. Improved natural killer cell function was also shown to improve within the same athlete during periods of greater intensity. This study, however, did not account for the change of season (summer versus winter) [14]. It appears that exercise must be intensive and extensive to provide a demonstrable protective effect among exercise subjects. In contrast to natural killer cells, exercise seems to decrease the functionality of an important innate immune system component–the neutrophil. Hack and colleagues [15] demonstrated a decrease in the phagocytic properties of neutrophils in athletes during periods of intensive activity compared with light activity. This effect has also been demonstrated in elite swimmers during times of intensive training. The oxidative activity of neutrophils was shown decrease in these athletes compared with age- and sex-matched sedentary control subjects [16]. It is evident that suppression of these effective phagocytes from intensive exercise plays a crucial role in respiratory disease potential. Studies of the adaptive immune system are not as clear in unveiling a direct relationship between exercise, URTI, and T- and B-cell response. T-cell function appears to be suppressed for several hours after high-intensity running [17]. A theorized mechanism of action relates to the change of T-cell activity with exposure to cortisol and epinephrine [18]. These findings, however, were not related to clinical expression of disease [1].

CANCER AND EXERCISE

Over 100 epidemiologic studies suggest that routine exercise is associated with a reduction of cancer, specifically colon and breast cancer [19]. Simple moderate activity such as mowing the lawn has shown a primary preventive protective benefit compared with activities of less intensity [20]. The evidence regarding secondary prevention is not as compelling but reveals some benefit associated with risk of death from breast cancer. Again, breast and colon cancer patients who exercise appear to decrease their relative risk (up to 40%) of cancer recurrence and cancer-related deaths. Although it appears that regular physical activity provides some protective benefit against cancer-related mortality and morbidity, additional large randomized controlled trials are necessary to fully uncover the specific mechanism of this beneficial observation in cancer patients.

AGING, GENDER, EXERCISE, AND IMMUNITY

As the body ages, disease is able to establish a foothold more easily than in the younger years. The body's innate ability to respond to and recover from foreign insult begins to waiver. A number of studies have revealed decreased T-cell response to pathogens in elderly subjects compared with young subjects [21,22]. It is difficult to isolate deconditioning from the ageing process as a primary cause of a dysfunctional immune system. This decrimental progression is known to be multifactorial in cause, including nutritional deficiencies, psychologic stress, and decreased cardiorespiratory condition. Despite this complex interaction leading to immune system dysfunction, recent studies demonstrate that regular physical activity in the elderly may enhance the immune system. Neimen and colleagues [23] randomized a group of elderly women (aged 67–85 years) to a walking protocol or to a calisthenic program for 12 weeks. Natural killer cell activity and T-cell function were used as end points in evaluating the potential effect of physical activity. Although there was a significant increase in cardiorespiratory condition in the walking group, there was no demonstrable benefit to immune function compared with the less active arm. Superior baseline cardiorespiratory condition seemed to benefit NCK activity and T-cell function and to prevent the occurrence of clinical infection compared with lower baseline cardiorespiratory condition. URTI was less prevalent in elderly participants who had a high baseline condition compared with the moderate exercise and calisthenic groups. No benefit was found with 12 weeks of moderate exercise in previously sedentary women.

IMMUNOLOGIC NUTRITIONAL CONCERNS

It has been proposed that nutrient supplementation may enhance the immune system, benefiting the transient immunosuppression seen from intensive training. This detrimental effect on the immune system may be related to the increased oxygen use during stressful activity, leading to the excessive production of free radical production. Therefore, research has been directed at antioxidatant therapy such as vitamin C and vitamin E. In addition, data have been collected regarding the effect of nutritional supplementation with betacarotene, zinc, iron, carbohydrate ingestion, and vitamins B_6 and B_{12}. Two South African studies have revealed encouraging results regarding vitamin C supplementation. One study analyzed athletes supplemented with 600 mg of vitamin C 3 weeks before a 90-km ultramarathon. These runners experienced fewer URTIs than nonsupplemented athletes during a 2-week period following the competition [24,25]. Results from additional studies evaluating high-dose supplementation have not been as promising as those for lower dose therapy and may create more gastrointestinal side effects. In contrast to vitamin C supplementation, treatment with excessive vitamin E and betacarotene appears to be detrimental to the immune system, increasing the oxidative stress on cells. This effect was demonstrated in a review of over 14,000 Scandinavian men supplemented with vitamin E and betacarotene, which increased their risk of URTIs while undergoing heavy exercise [26]. Several studies have also examined the function and levels of minerals in exercising subjects. Particular research has focused on zinc, iron, and glutamate supplementation and their effects in athletes. There is no compelling research recommending specific preventive therapy for certain elements. Iron deficiency appears to have little effect on antibody generation, whereas research is conflicting regarding its effect on cell-mediated immunity. Small studies on glutamine supplementation showed no benefit in enhancing immune cell levels or function in exercising patients [27]; however, it is known that excessive intake can have a deleterious effect on the immune system [28]. At present, athletes should obtain their nutritional supplementation from a well-rounded diet. In addition, taking a simple multivitamin is prudent because there is no evidence that this will cause excessive vitamin or mineral levels in the body. Training with optimal stores of carbohydrate not only appears to provide the necessary fuel for activity but also seems to negate some of the immunosuppressive effects of exercise. One study indicated that carbohydrate ingestion positively influenced blood cortisol, lymphocyte counts, and natural killer cell activity during the exercise recovery period [29]. No analysis of clinical disease relationship was evaluated in this study. Overall, good dietary carbohydrate replacement that matches the training session appears to support and boost the immune system.

SUMMARY

What does this mean for one's patients? All patients must be considered athletes because everyone undergoes various stressors of daily living that most likely affect the immune system in ways similar to intensive exercise. We must continue to appreciate the impact of stress and the environment on immune system function. When counseling patients, attention should be given to that patient's mental, social, and physical stress levels. It is prudent that emphasis be given to the role of moderately intensive exercise and nutrition as part of a comprehensive prevention program.

References

[1] Nieman DC. Risk of upper respiratory tract infection in athletes: an epidemiologic and immunologic perspective. J Athl Train 1997;32(4):344–9.

[2] Delhagen K, Miller B. Running from colds. Runner's World 1990;25:18–21.

[3] Adams PF, Benson V. Current estimates form the National Health Interview Survey, 1990. National Center for Health Statistics. Vital Health Stat 1991;10(181):1–212.

[4] Simon HD. The immunology of exercise, a brief review. JAMA 1984;252:2735–8.

[5] Medical physiology. In: Rhoades RA, Tanner GA, editors. The immune system. Little, Brown, and Company: Boston; 1995. p. 220–4.

[6] Haynes BF, Gauci AS. Harrison's principles of internal medicine. In: Fauci AS, Braunwald E, Isselbacher K, et al, editors. Disorders of the immune system, connective tissue, and joints. McGraw-Hill: New York; 1998. p. 1753–72.

[7] Goronzy JJ, Weyand CM. Cecil Textbook of Medicine. Arends WP, Armitage JO, Drazen JM, et al, editors. 22nd edition. The innate and adaptive immune systems. W.B. Saunders: Philadelphia, PA; 2004. p. 161–5.

[8] Pershin BB, Geliev AB, Tolstov DV, et al. Reactions of immune system to physical exercises. Russ J Immunol 2003;7(1):1–20.

[9] Mackinnon LT, Chick TW, As AV, et al. The effect of exercise on secretory and natural immunity. Adv Exp Med Biol 1987;216A:869–76.

[10] Fahlman MM, Engels HJ. Mucosal IgA and URTI in American college football players: a longitudinal study. Med Sci Sports Exerc 2005;37(3):374–80.

[11] Novas AP, Rowbottom DG, Jenkins DG. Tennis, incidence of URTI and salivary IgA. Int J Sports Med 2003;24(3):223–9.

[12] Klentrou P, Cieslak T, MacNeil M, et al. Effect of moderate exercise on salivary immunoglobulin A and infection risk in humans. Eur J Appl Physiol 2002;87:153–8.

[13] Nieman DC, Buckley KS, Henson DA, et al. Immune function in marathon runners versus sedentary controls. Med Sci Sports Exerc 1995;27:986–92.

[14] Tvede N, Steensberg J, Baslund B, et al. Cellular immunity in highly-trained elite racing cyclists and controls during periods of training with high and low intensity. Scand J Med Sci Sports 1991;1:163–6.

[15] Hack V, Strobel G, Weiss M, et al. PMN cell counts and phagocytic activity of highly trained athletes depend on training period. J Appl Physiol 1944;77:1731–5.

[16] Pyne DB, Baker MS, Fricker PA, et al. Effects of an intensive 12-wk training program by elite swimmers on neutrophil oxidative activity. Med Sci Sports Exerc 1995;27:536–42.

[17] Nieman DC, Simandle S, Henson DA, et al. Lymphocyte proliferative response. Int J Sports Med 1995;16:404–9.

[18] Crary B, Borysenko M, Sutherland DC, et al. Decrease in mitogen responsiveness of mononuclear cells from peripheral blood after epinephrine administration in humans. J Immunol 1983;130:694–9.

[19] Haydon AM, Macinnis R, English D, et al. The effect of physical activity and body size on survival after diagnosis with colorectal cancer. Gut 2005;1:62–7.

[20] Lee IM. Physical activity and cancer prevention—data from epidemiologic studies. Med Sci Sports Exerc 2003;35:1823–7.
[21] Canonica GW, Ciprandi G, Caria M, et al. Defect of autologous mixed lymphocyte reaction and interleukin-2 in aged individuals. Mech Ageing Dev 1985;32:205–12.
[22] Krishanaraj R, Blandford G. Age-associated alterations in human natural killer cells. Increased activity as per conventional and kinetic analysis. Clin Immunol Immunopathol 1987;45:268–85.
[23] Nieman DC, Henson DA, Gusewitch G, et al. Physical activity and immune function in elderly women. Med Sci Sports Exerc 1993;25(7):823–31.
[24] Peters IM, Bateman ED. Ultramarathon running and upper respiratory tract infections. S Afr Med J 1983;64:582–4.
[25] Peters EM, Goetzsche JM, Grobbelarr B, et al. Vitamin C supplementation reduces the incidence of postrace symptoms of upper respiratory tract infections in ultramarathon runners. Am J Clin Nutr 1993;57:170–4.
[26] Hemila H, Virtamo J, Albanes D, et al. Physical activity and the common cold in men administered vitamin E and beta carotene. Med Sci Sports Exerc 2003;35(11):1815–20.
[27] Krzywkowski K, Petersen EW, Ostrowski K, et al. Effect of glutamine supplementation on exercise-induced changes in lymphocyte function. Am J Physiol 2001;281:1259–65.
[28] Speich M, Pineau A, Ballereau F. Minerals, trace elements and related biological variables in athletes and during physical activity. Clin Chim Acta 2001;312(1,2):1–11.
[29] Henson DA, Nieman DC, Blodgett AD, et al. Influence of exercise mode and carbohydrate on the immune response to prolonged exercise. Int J Sport Nutr 1999;9:213–28.

Clin Sports Med 26 (2007) 321–344

CLINICS IN SPORTS MEDICINE

ELSEVIER
SAUNDERS

Prevention of Infectious Diseases in Athletes

Anthony Luke, MD, MPH[a],*, Pierre d'Hemecourt, MD[b]

[a]Departments of Orthopaedic Surgery and Family and Community Medicine,
Primary Care Sports Medicine, University of California San Francisco, 500 Parnassus Ave.,
MU-320W, San Francisco, CA 94143-0728, USA
[b]Primary Care Sports Medicine, Harvard University, Children's Hospital of Boston,
319 Longwood Ave., Boston, MA 02115, USA

Infections in sports can be serious medical problems. They can affect individual athletes, resulting in morbidity and decreased performance [1]. They can also be spread to other athletes, putting them at risk for similar disease and complications. The sports medicine physician may face challenging issues regarding infectious diseases when dealing with teams or highly competitive athletes who have difficulties taking time off to recover. One must treat the individual sick athlete and take the necessary precautions to contain the spread of communicable disease to the surrounding team, staff, relatives, and other contacts.

The authors aim to translate recommendations in public health to practice in a sports medicine setting. Sports physicians have an opportunity to see athletes during adolescence and adulthood who might not come in for routine health maintenance except when related to their sports. Primary prevention of infectious disease, the ideal goal, deals with avoiding the development of the disease before infection occurs. Immunizations are an example of primary prevention and have been the most successful public health programs for disease prophylaxis. Secondary prevention for infection control involves prevention of spread to others. Athletes are often exposed to many different people, travel to compete in various environments locally and internationally, and engage in higher-risk activities, often in close contact with others [2]. The authors discuss the preventive strategies for infectious disease in sport, including (1) a review of immunization recommendations and prophylaxis guidelines, (2) improvements in personal hygiene and prevention of spread of infectious organisms by direct contact, (3) insect-borne disease precautions, and (4) prevention of sexually transmitted diseases (STDs). A special emphasis on immunizations focuses on pertussis, influenza, and meningococcal prophylaxis.

*Corresponding author. E-mail address: lukea@orthosurg.ucsf.edu (A. Luke).

0278-5919/07/$ – see front matter
doi:10.1016/j.csm.2007.04.006

PUBLIC HEALTH, INFECTIOUS DISEASES, AND SPORTS

Public health plays an insidious role in our everyday lives to keep individuals safe from communicable diseases, accidents, environmental concerns, and countless other dangers. Programs are most successful when a disease no longer becomes a worry for the population through active prevention strategies. Much of our understanding comes from history and from recognizing the imminent dangers so we can prevent diseases from occurring the next time.

Medical reports from major athletic events provide examples of issues that can be encountered by the sports medicine physician. Mass-gathering events, such as the Olympics, highlight some of the concerns that can occur with sports and infectious diseases. International athletes compete together from countries with different endemic microorganisms and variable health care practices. For example, an outbreak of measles occurred in a Special Olympics event in St. Paul, Minnesota. The point of infection was suspected to be a track and field athlete from Argentina, resulting in measles infections in 16 individuals from 7 different states [3]. An outbreak of influenza that occurred during the 1988 Calgary Olympics was believed to have possibly affected the performances of some athletes [4]. The pneumococcal vaccine was recommended to athletes before competing in the 1992 Barcelona Olympics because of resistant *Streptococcus pneumoniae* strains endemic in Spain [5]. Medical reporting and surveillance of infections are extremely important to attempt to contain spread of disease. At the 1996 Atlanta Olympics, a priority of surveillance was to identify unusual presentations and infectious disease outbreaks to actively implement same-day medical and public health interventions [6].

It is an important responsibility of physicians to report specific infectious diseases, especially if an outbreak is suspected (Box 1) [7]. Health professionals should contact their local public health officer to determine whether other cases are occurring and what precautions need to be taken in the event of a serious outbreak. In the past few years, infections such as severe acute respiratory syndrome [8] have required the need of quarantine to help control the spread of these dangerous diseases. Health care professionals should report all clinically significant adverse events following immunization to the Vaccine Adverse Events Reporting System [9].

ATHLETES ARE "HIGHER RISK"

The risk of disease transmission depends on the infectious agent—for example, whether it is spread by way of respiratory secretions, skin contact, or blood. In the context of infections spread by aerosol droplets, "close contact" can mean caring for or living with an infected patient or having a high likelihood of direct contact with the respiratory secretions or body fluids of an infected patient. Examples of close contact include kissing or embracing, sharing eating or drinking utensils, talking to someone within 3 ft, physical examination, and any other direct physical contact between people. Close contact does not include activities such as walking by a person or briefly sitting across from someone [10].

Box 1: Infectious diseases designated as notifiable at the national level during 2004

Acquired immunodeficiency syndrome (AIDS)

Anthrax

Botulism

Brucellosis

Chancrodi

Chlamydia trachomatis, genital infection

Cholera

Coccidioidomycosis

Cryptosproidiososis

Cryptosporidiosis

Cyclosporiasis

Diphtheria

Ehrlichiosis

   Human granulocytic

   Human monocytic

   Human, other or unspecified agent

Encephalitis/meningitis, arboviral

   California serogroup

   Eastern equine

   Powassan

   St. Louis

   Western equine

   West Nile

Enterohemorrhagic *Escherichia coli* (EHEC)

   EHEC O157:H7

   EHEC Shiga toxin-positive, serogroup non-O157

   EHEC Shiga toxin-positive, not serogrouped

Giardiasis

Gonorrhea

Haemophilus influenzae, invasive disease

Hansen disease (leprosy)

Hantavirus pulmonary syndrome

Hemolytic uremic syndrome, postdiarrheal

Hepatitis A, viral, acute

Hepatitis B, viral, acute

Box 1: (continued)

Hepatitis B, viral, chronic

Hepatitis B, perinatal infection

Hepatitis C, acute

Hepatitis C, virus infection (past or present)

Human immunodeficiency virus (HIV) infection

    Adult (age ≥13 years)

    Pediatric (age <13 years)

Influenza-associated pediatric mortality[a]

Legionellosis

Listeriosis

Lyme disease

Malaria

Measles

Meningococcal disease

Mumps

Pertussis

Plague

Poliomyelitis, paralytic

Psittacosis

Q fever

Rabies

    Animal

    Human

Rocky Mountain spotted fever

Rubella

Rubella, congenital syndrome

Salmonellosis

Severe acute respiratory syndrome–associated coronavirus (SARS-CoV) disease

Shigellosis

Smallpox[a]

Streptococcal disease, invasive, group A

Streptococcal toxic-shock syndrome

Streptococcus pneumoniae, invasive disease

    Drug-resistant, all ages

    Age <5 years

Syphilis

Syphilis, congenital

Box 1: (*continued*)

Tetanus

Toxic-shock syndrome (other than streptococcal)

Trichinellosis[b]

Tuberculosis

Tularemia

Typhoid fever

Vancomycin-intermediate *Staphylococcus aureus* infection (VISA)[c]

Vancomycin-resistant *Staphylococcus aureus* infection (VRSA)[c]

Varicella

Varicella deaths

Yellow fever

[a]New for 2004, as of October 4, 2004.
[b]Formerly referred to as trichinosis.
[c]New for 2004, as of January 1, 2004.

From Jajosky RA, Hall PA, Adams DA, et al. Summary of notifiable diseases—United States, 2004. MMWR Morb Mortal Wkly Rep 2006;53(53):1–79.

Athletes may share personal items (eg, towels, water bottles, and soap) and equipment (eg, weights). They may live in dormitories or in hotel rooms while traveling, which leads to close contact and high exposure to teammates. They participate in higher-risk activities [2,11]. Fewer athletes practice safe sex, which can lead to STDs in homosexual and in heterosexual individuals. Athletes also use more illicit drugs and alcohol, which can place them at risk of intravenous needle exposure [12,13]. Steroids, hormones, and vitamins are other substances that some athletes are injecting [14,15]. Tattoos are popular among athletes, which are another source of needle infection risk.

IMMUNIZATIONS

Active immunization involves the administration of all or part of a microorganism or a modified product of that microorganism, such as an antigen or protein. This administration stimulates an immune response to develop protection against future exposure to the infection [16]. Although most vaccines are over 90% effective, they are not guaranteed to promote immune protection [16].

Immunizations typically involve inactivated vaccines or live, attenuated viruses. Inactivated vaccines include killed virus or bacterial proteins to stimulate one's immune system to develop antibodies to any similar virus or bacteria. More side effects are associated with the live, attenuated viruses–typically local pain and, rarely, hypersensitivity reactions to vaccine constituents. A mild febrile illness, a recent exposure to an infectious disease, pregnancy, breastfeeding, nonspecific allergies, and family history of an adverse event after immunization, including seizures, are NOT contraindications for immunization [16].

Sports medicine physicians need to consider the following indications for immunizations (Tables 1 and 2): (1) routine health maintenance; (2) catch-up immunizations for failed or missed immunizations; (3) immunizations of high risk groups (ie, splenectomy, chronic disease, immunocompromised); (4) travel to an endemic area; (5) close contact with an infected individual, or (6) recent potential exposure to an infectious agent.

When doing preparticipation physical examinations, it is sometimes assumed that athletes have received all their immunizations. Proof of immunizations is required by schools and colleges, although exceptions can be given to individuals refusing to receive immunizations. In a study surveying 69,115 Minnesota children who entered kindergarten in 1992, by 19 months of age, 73% of students had received the measles, mumps, and rubella (MMR) vaccine, and only 39% had received their fourth dose of diphtheria, tetanus, and pertussis vaccine (DTaP) [17]. Vaccination rates can vary substantially by age, race/ethnicity, and neighborhood [17]. White, non-Hispanic students usually have higher vaccination rates than children of other racial/ethnic groups. It has been estimated that 79% of whites, 76% of Hispanics, and 71% of African Americans are fully immunized [18].

Measles, Mumps, and Rubella

Although MMR vaccines have been administered for many decades and incidences of disease are presently low [7], the diseases can still occur in the adult population. Between 1986 and 1989, 6% of the measles cases occurred in college

Table 1
Routine immunizations for adults recommended by the Centers for Disease Control and Prevention, October 2006–September 2007

Vaccine	Age group (y)		
	19–49	50–64	≥65
Tetanus, diptheria, pertussis (Td/DTaP)	1-dose Td booster every 10 y Substitute 1 dose of DTaP for Td		
Human papilloma virus (HPV)	3 doses (female patients)		
Measles, mumps, rubella (MMR)	1 or 2 doses	1 dose	
Varicella	2 doses (0, 4–8 wk)	2 doses (0, 4–8 wk)	
Influenza	1 dose annually	1 dose annually	
Pneumococcal (polysaccharide)	1–2 doses		1 dose
Hepatitis A	2 doses (0, 6–12 mo or 0, 6–18 mo)		
Hepatitis B	3 doses (0, 1–2, 4–6 mo)		
Meningococcal	1 or more doses		

Data from United States Department of Health and Human Services, Centers for Disease Control and Prevention. Recommended adult immunization schedule, by vaccine and age group. Available at http://www.cdc.gov/vaccines/recs/schedules/downloads/adult/06-07/adult-schedule-11x17.pdf; Accessed November 30, 2006.

Table 2
Catch-up immunization schedule for children aged 7 through 18 years recommended by the Centers for Disease Control and Prevention

Vaccine	Minimum interval between doses		
	Dose 1 to dose 2	Dose 2 to dose 3	Dose 3 to booster dose
Tetanus, diptheria (Td)[h]	4 wk	6 mo	6 mo if first dose given at age <12 mo and current age <11 y, otherwise 5 y
Inactivated poliovirus (IPV)[b,i]	4 wk	4 wk	IPV[b,i]
Hepatitis B (HepB)[c]	4 wk	8 wk (and 16 wk after first dose)	
Measles, mumps, rubella (MMR)[d]	4 wk		
Varicella[i]	4 wk		

[a]DTaP. The fifth dose is not necessary if the fourth dose was administered after the fourth birthday.

[b]IPV. For children who received an all-IPV or all-oral poliovirus (OPV) series, a fourth dose is not necessary if a third was administered at age ≥4 years. If OPV and IPV were administered as part of a series, then a total of four doses should be given, regardless of the child's current age.

[c]HepB. Administer the three-dose series to all children and adolescents <19 years of age if they were not previously vaccinated.

[d]MMR. The second dose of MMR is recommended routinely at age 4 to 6 years but may be administered earlier if desired.

[e]Hib. Vaccine is not generally recommended for children aged ≥5 years.

[f]Hib. If current age <12 months and the first 2 doses were Haemophilus b conjugate vaccine (PRP-OMP) (pedvaxHIB or ComVax [Merck]), then the third (and final) dose should be administered at age 12 to 15 months and at least 8 weeks after the second dose.

[g]PCV. Vaccine is not generally recommended for children aged ≥5 years.

[h]Td. Adolescent tetanus, diptheria, and pertussis vaccine (DTaP) may be substituted for any dose in a primary catch-up series or as a booster if age appropriate for DTaP. A 5-year interval from the last Td dose is encouraged when DTaP is used as a booster dose. See ACIP recommendations for further information.

[i]IPV. Vaccine is not generally recommended for persons aged ≥18 years.

[j]Varicella. Administer the two-dose series to all susceptible adolescents aged ≥13 years.

Data from United States Department of Health and Human Services, Centers for Disease Control and Prevention. 2007 Child & Adolescent Immunization Schedules. Available at http://www.cdc.gov/vaccines/recs/schedules/downloads/child/2007/child-schedule-color-print.pdf; Accessed November 30, 2006.

students [19]. Enzyme-linked immunosorbent assay tests for antibodies to MMR are available to detect for immunization status [19]. In a series of 256 students, 53 (21%) were found to be seronegative to measles alone, 13 (5%) were seronegative to rubella alone, and 5 (2%) were seronegative to measles and rubella. Eighty-six percent of the individuals seronegative to measles had previously received a dose of measles vaccine. Following a second injection, conversion to seropositive status rose to 97% and 100% for measles and rubella, respectively. These data support the need for a two-dose vaccine schedule [19].

Pneumococcal Vaccine

Pneumococcal vaccine is administered to prevent *Streptococcus pneumoniae* infections. A conjugate heptavalent is given to during the first 2 years of life. A polysaccharide vaccine is provided to high-risk individuals older than 2 years against 23 types of *Streptococcus pneumonia* that account for 90% of invasive disease [20]. High-risk groups include patients who have asplenia, sickle cell disease, diabetes mellitus, cirrhosis, immunocompromised states, chronic cardiac or pulmonary disease, or age 65 years or older. Immunity following vaccination is successful for periods of 5 to 10 years, requiring booster injections [20].

Hepatitis B

Hepatitis B is a blood-borne virus transmitted through sexual contact and parenteral exposure to blood and blood components [14]. Hepatitis B has a greater risk for transmission in sports than HIV. The risk of HIV transmission is estimated to between 1 in 1 million games and 1 in 85 million games [14,21]. The risk arises if bleeding and skin exudates from an infected individual come into contact with open wounds in another athlete, particularly during contact and collision sports. There are no confirmed cases of spread of HIV through sports [14]; however, 5 out of 10 high school sumo wrestlers at one club developed hepatitis B [22]. Another case series reported on 11 of 65 American football players who developed hepatitis B over a period of 19 months [23]. Contact through open wounds, cuts, and abrasions were the suspected routes of transmission.

Primary prevention

Although hepatitis A is a considered immunization in athletes who are traveling to endemic areas, routine vaccination for hepatitis B is recommended for all individuals after birth using single or combination vaccines [24]. A three-dose immunization schedule is typically used after 18 years of age, with injections at 0 months, 1 month, and 6 months, although there is an optional four-dose schedule [25]. The licensed vaccines have had 90% to 95% efficacy of preventing hepatitis B, with immunity lasting 15 years or longer [25]. Immunizations for hepatitis B should be checked during the preparticipation physical examination, and catch-up immunizations recommended to the individual (see Table 2). If individuals are uncertain about their immunization status, serologic testing for antibody to hepatitis B surface antigen can determine immunity.

Secondary prevention

When athletes are known to be infected with hepatitis B, secondary prevention includes education on personal hygiene, appropriate management of open wounds, proper use of protective equipment, safe sex practices using a condom, and avoidance of intravenous blood transmission (eg, through needle sharing and illicit drug use).

Pertussis, Tetanus, and Polio

Bordetella pertussis, which is responsible for whooping cough, is a gram-negative coccobacillus transmitted by way of airborne droplets [26]. Although tetanus and polio have been controlled well with the use of vaccines [7], the rate of pertussis cases has been increasing in adolescents and adults despite routine immunizations [27]. Most cases occur in patients 10 years or older [28].

The infection is most concerning for infants because immunity is not complete until older ages. The spread to infants is typically from adults. Pertussis usually presents with nonspecific upper respiratory tract infection symptoms for 1 to 2 weeks (catarrhal stage), after which the paroxysmal and sometimes uncontrollable cough develops [26]. The cough is not necessarily always followed by the classic "whooping" sound, and pertussis should be considered with any persistent, prolonged cough.

Primary prevention
The whole-cell pertussis vaccine is estimated to be approximately 85% effective [29]. This vaccine is still recommended for use in the routine immunization of young children; however, the immunity provided begins to decline at 4 to 12 years following vaccination, which makes adolescents and adults susceptible [27]. Rare adverse reactions from the vaccine include hypotonic, hyporesponsive episodes, high fever, seizures, and anaphylaxis [26]. Two acellular vaccines have been introduced that are as effective as whole-cell vaccines and have fewer adverse reactions [30]. These vaccines are combined with tetanus toxoid and reduced diphtheria toxoid (DTaP). The Centers for Disease Control and Prevention (CDC) recommends use of these DTaP boosters rather than the tetanus-diptheria (Td) booster starting after 11 to 12 years of age [31].

Secondary prevention
For pertussis, individuals are most contagious during the first 1 to 2 weeks during the catarrhal stage but should be considered contagious until 3 weeks after the paroxysmal stage ends or after taking antibiotics for 5 days [32]. Diagnosis of pertussis infection is best performed through polymerase chain reaction assay (sensitivity, 94%; specificity, 97%) or through direct fluorescent antibody testing (sensitivity, 52%; specificity, 98%). Nasal swab cultures (sensitivity, 15%; specificity, 100%) are routinely performed; however, they have high false negative rates and take 7 to 12 days to yield results [33]. Physicians in the United States are legally required to report cases of pertussis to state public health departments [26]. It is estimated that 80% of susceptible household contacts will be infected after close contact [26]. Antibiotic prophylaxis is recommended for close contacts of persons who have pertussis to prevent outbreaks [34]. Preferred drugs are azithromycin for 5 days, clarithromycin for 7 days, or trimethoprim-sulfamethoxazole or erythromycin for 14 days, which are similar for prophylaxis and treatment [34].

Influenza
Influenza presents with constitutional symptoms of fever, chills, malaise, fatigue, and myalgia in addition to upper respiratory tract symptoms of a sore throat, cough, and rhinitis. Rarely, more serious conditions can occur, including encephalopathy, transverse myelitis, myocarditis, and pericarditis [9]. Immunogenicity is determined by hemaglutinins and neuraminidases on the virus surface. Antigenic drift can occur that can mutate the virus into different

strains. Transmission occurs by way of respiratory droplets. The virus has an incubation period of usually 2 days (range, 1–4 days), and adults are infectious from the day before symptoms begin to approximately 5 days after the illness starts [9]. Symptoms usually last a week, although less likely, symptoms can last longer than 2 weeks. These symptoms can be very disruptive for treatment and challenging for the athlete to keep training and competing. A case series of 81 students, mostly healthy adolescents at a ski school in Austria, reported a severe outbreak of influenza A, leading to an attack rate of 49%, with 69% becoming ill within 2 days of the outbreak. Two students were hospitalized with pneumonia and 1 died [35].

Primary prevention

Influenza vaccines contain strains of antigenically equivalent strains of influenza similar to those annually recommended: influenza A (H3N2), influenza A (H1N1), and a B virus. Depending on the emergence and spread of new strains, other virus strains can be added to update the vaccine [9]. The efficacy of influenza vaccine is approximately 70% to 90% for individuals under age 65 years [36]. Vaccination for influenza should occur in the fall (October or November), at the beginning of the flu season (Box 2) [9]. Antibodies develop approximately 2 weeks after vaccination [9,37].

Inactivated influenza vaccine is generally appropriate for all populations requiring influenza vaccine. Three influenza vaccines were available in the United States for the 2006 to 2007 season: Fluzone (manufactured by Sanofi-Pasteur); Fluvirin (manufactured by Novartis); and Fluarix (manufactured by GlaxoSmithKline). The typical dose is 0.5 mL administered intramuscularly, usually in the deltoid muscle. Live, attenuated influenza vaccine (LAIV) is approved for use in healthy, nonpregnant individuals aged 5 to 49

Box 2: Indications for influenza vaccine

1. Adults and children with chronic disorders of the cardiorespiratory system, including asthma

2. Adults and children who have chronic disease which may require regular medical follow-up or hospitalization, including immunodeficiency

3. Young children aged 6–23 months

4. Children aged 6 months to 18 years on long-term aspirin therapy and at risk for Reye's syndrome

5. Persons aged >65 years

6. Residents of nursing homes or chronic-care facilities

7. Health care workers

8. Travelers to influenza-endemic areas

Adapted from Smith NM, Bresee JS, Shay DK, et al. Prevention and control of influenza: recommendations of the Advisory Committee on Immunization Practices (ACIP). MMWR Recomm Rep 2006;55(RR-10):1–42.

years. The LAIV is administered by way of a nasal spray once in each nostril (FluMist, manufactured by MedImmune). Individuals who have a hypersensitivity or anaphylactic reaction to components of the flu vaccine or to eggs should not be vaccinated [9].

Adults reported having a 19% reduction in severe febrile illnesses after LAIV compared with placebo [38]. Side effects from LAIV increased in adults within 7 days of immunization compared with placebo and consisted mainly of nasal congestion (44.5% versus 27.1%) and sore throat (27.8% versus 17.1%), which lasted, on average, 2 days. Less common complaints were tiredness, cough, and chills. There was no significant difference in the number of mild febrile illnesses between immunization and placebo groups [39]. Injections can be scheduled to occur at the optimum time during the athlete's competitive schedule to minimize concern about side effects.

When inactivated influenza vaccine shortages occurred in previous years, the vaccine was recommended for high-risk groups as priority; however, the general recommendation now is to offer the immunization annually to anyone who wishes to reduce the likelihood of being ill with influenza or transmitting the virus if they should become infected [9]. Although this policy cannot be directly translated into a benefit for the athlete, depending on the level of athlete, the use of the LAIV may also be beneficial to prevent lost time from sport. Influenza vaccine has been suggested for competitive athletes and essential personnel, especially before international events occurring during the influenza season [4,40].

Secondary prevention

Treatment with antiviral medications can reduce the duration of uncomplicated influenza A and B illness by approximately 1 day when administered within 2 days of illness onset [41,42]. Recommended antiviral treatment should be given for 5 days [9]. Four antiviral agents are currently available: amantadine, rimantadine, zanamivir, and oseltamivir [9]. The influenza A virus, however, has become resistant to amantadine and rimantadine, which are presently not recommended to be used as first-line drugs [43]. Zanamivir (Ralenza, dry powder taken by orally inhaled route) and oseltamivir (Tamiflu, capsule or oral suspension) are neuraminidase inhibitors and can be used to treat patients and to control influenza outbreaks in closed settings. Although typically used in nursing homes, an outbreak in a dormitory may require chemoprophylaxis [9]. There are limited data to suggest that serious complications from influenza, such as lower respiratory tract infections, may be reduced [44]. The use of antiviral medications for prophylaxis of influenza is unclear and is not yet recommended for routine seasonal control [45]. The use of oseltamivir, however, has been recommended in specific cases, especially if there is high risk of spread such as household contacts and if individuals have not been immunized [46]. Oseltamivir was used to treat 36 of 188 patients, including 13 athletes during the 2002 Salt Lake City Winter Olympics, with medications given to close contacts, which was believed to limit the spread of influenza [47].

Clinical history and physical examination are still the mainstays for diagnosing influenza. Rapid swab tests are available and take approximately 30 minutes to detect the influenza virus. The tests are less sensitive (72%–95%) and specific (76%–86%) than the traditional viral cultures [48]. They have moderate sensitivities for influenza antigens and are more likely to produce false negative rather than false positive results [48,49]. Direct and indirect fluorescent antibody staining tests are also available, but they are ordered more in hospitals because they take 2 to 4 hours to obtain results [49]. Viral cultures are still the "gold standard" for confirming the presence of influenza and identifying the strains and subtypes [9].

Meningitis

Neisseria meningitides is a serious concern, especially for the adolescent and college populations. An alarming trend during the 1970s demonstrated an increase in meningitis deaths in college students, with living in dormitories being a risk factor. The disease can be spread by asymptomatic carriers. Students living in dormitories were 9 to 23 times more likely of getting infected than those living in other types of accommodations [50]. Freshmen who lived in dormitories had an elevated risk of meningococcal disease (odds ratio, 3.6; 95% confidence interval, 1.6–8.5; $P = .003$) compared with other college students [51]. Aside from the risk of death, 11% to 19% of survivors of meningitis have serious sequelae such as neurologic disability, limb loss, and hearing loss [50].

Primary prevention

Routine vaccination with meningococcal vaccine is recommended for college freshmen living in dormitories and for other populations at increased risk. The CDC Advisory Committee on Immunization Practices recommends routine vaccination of young adolescents (11–12 years old) with meningococcal vaccine (MCV4) at the preadolescent health care visit [50]. Therefore, sports medicine physicians may be faced with higher frequency of checking for meningococcal immunization status for high school and college athletes. A tetravalent conjugate vaccine (Menactra, Sanofi Pasteur) is available against *Neisseria meningitidis* isolates A, C, Y, and W-135 in a 0.5-mL single-dose vial. Over the age of 11 years, 75% of the meningococcal infections are caused by strains C, Y, or W-135 (CDC, unpublished data, 2004) [50]. Another vaccine, Menomune (Aventis Pasteur Limited), has been licensed since 1981 and has a similar immunogenicity profile to Menactra and is delivered subcutaneously as a 0.5-mL dose. Menactra and Menomune have serum bactericidal protection ranging from 89.4% and 94.4% for strain W-135 and 73.5% and 79.4% for strain Y, respectively [50]. Revaccination may be necessary for individuals at high risk after 5 years [52,53]. Common side effects with MCV4 were local pain in just over 50% of patients, followed by swelling, induration, and redness in approximately 10.8% to 17.1%. Fever was reported in 5.1% of children 18 years old or younger and in 1.5% of adults [50].

Secondary prevention
Close contacts are at high risk and should be treated with chemoprophylaxis ideally within 24 hours of identifying the index patient [50]. The goal of treatment is to reduce nasopharyngeal carriage of *N meningitidis*. After more than 14 days after the onset of illness in the index patient, chemoprophylaxis is not necessary [50]. A single dose of ciprofloxacin (500 mg orally) or ceftriaxone (250 mg by intramuscular injection), or rifampin (600 mg twice a day for 2 days) is recommended for adults. Children between 1 month and 18 years old may take rifampin (10 mg/kg every 12 hours for 2 days), or ceftriaxone (125 mg intramuscularly) if younger than 15 years [50]. One dose of azithromycin (500 mg) was also shown to eradicate *N meningitidis* and may represent another treatment option [54].

Human Papillomavirus
Human papillomavirus (HPV) is associated with 99% of cervical cancers and anogenital, head and neck, and nonmelanoma skin cancers. It is an STD and can be diagnosed by abnormal cervical cell changes seen on Pap smear [55]. This is a common infection, especially in sexually active adolescents and university students [56].

Primary prevention
Primary prevention is now possible with two new vaccines: a bivalent vaccine against HPV types 16 and 18 and a quadravalent vaccine against types 6, 11, 16, and 18. The vaccines have a three-dose schedule: 0, 1, and 6 months (bivalent vaccine) and 0, 2, and 6 months (quadravalent vaccine). At 4.5 years, the bivalent vaccine was effective for producing a persistent antibody response against HPV 16 and 18, with more than 98% seropositivity and 96.9% effectiveness (95% confidence interval, 81.3–99.9) in reducing the number of reported abnormalities on Pap smear, colposcopy, or both [57]. Routine vaccination with three doses of quadrivalent HPV vaccine is recommended for girls 11 to 12 years old but can be started in girls as young as 9 years. Girls and women aged 13 to 26 years who have not been vaccinated previously or who have not completed the full vaccine series are recommended to receive a catch-up series. The vaccine is intended to be administered before potential exposure to HPV through sexual contact [58].

Secondary prevention
Secondary prevention involves checking the affected individual's partners for signs of genital warts and other STDs. Regular cervical screen is recommended. Use of condoms and education on spread is important. HPV infection persists for life; however, the degree and duration of contagiousness is yet unknown [59].

Travel Immunizations
Athletes traveling need to consider the endemic diseases in the geographic location where they are competing. They should be aware of risks of acquiring common diseases, their accommodations (urban versus rural), local foods, and

customs. Immunizations should ideally be planned 4 or more months in advance to allow for adequate time to administer vaccines (Table 3). There are many resources for information about prevention of infectious diseases for travelers (Table 4).

Table 3
Recommended immunizations for travelers to developing countries[a]

	Length of travel		
Immunizations	Brief, <2 wk	Intermediate, 2 wk to 3 mo	Long-term residential, >3 mo
Review and complete age-appropriate childhood schedule (see text for details) DTaP, poliovirus, pneumococcal, and Haemophilus influenzae type b vaccines may be given at 4-wk intervals if necessary to complete the recommended schedule before departure Measles: 2 additional doses given if younger than 12 mo of age at first dose Varicella Hepatitis B[b]	+	+	+
Yellow fever[c]	+	+	+
Hepatitis A[d]	+	+	+
Typhoid fever[e]	±	+	+
Meningococcal disease[f]	±	±	±
Rabies[g]	±	+	+
Japanese encephalitis[h]	±	±	+

+ = recommended; ± = consider.

[a]See disease-specific chapters in Section 3 of the AAP Red Book for details: [Red Book: 2006 report of the Committee of Infectious Diseases. 27th edition. Elk Grove Village, (IL) American Academy of Pediatrics; 2006]. For further sources of information, see text.

[b]If insufficient time to complete 6-month primary series, accelerated series can be given (see text for details).

[c]For regions with endemic infection.

[d]Indicated for travelers to areas with intermediate or high endemic rates of HAV infection.

[e]Indicated for travelers who will consume food and liquids in areas of poor sanitation.

[f]Recommended for regions of Africa with endemic infection and during local epidemics, and required for travel to Saudi Arabia for the Hajj.

[g]Indicated for people with high risk of animal exposure (especially to dogs) and for travelers to countries with endemic infection.

[h]For regions with endemic infection. For high-risk activities in areas experiencing outbreaks, vaccine is recommended, even for brief travel.

From American Academy of Pediatrics. International travel. In: Pickering LK, editor. Red book: 2006 report of the committee on infectious diseases. 27th edition. Elk Grove Village (IL): American Academy of Pediatrics; 2006. p. 99; with permission from the American Academy of Pediatrics.

Table 4
More common tick-borne diseases

Tick-borne disease	Organism	Common vector (geographic area)
Rocky Mountain spotted fever	*Rickettsia rickettsii*	Dog tick, *Dermacentor variabilis* (central, Pacific coastal, and eastern US) Rocky Mountain wood tick, *Dermacentor andersoni* (western US)
Human monocytotropic ehrlichiosis	*Ehrlichia chaffeensis*	Lone Star tick (south central US in Maryland, Arkansas, Tennessee, Oklahoma, and Missouri) [60]
Human granulocytotropic anaplasmosis	*Anaplasma phagocytophilum*	Blacklegged tick, *Ixodes scapularis* (north central US and New England) *Ixodes pacificus* (California) [75]
Lyme disease	*Borrelia burgdorferi*	*Ixodes scapularis* (eastern US in New England and mid-Atlantic states and Midwest US in Wisconsin and Minnesota) *Ixodes pacificus* (west in northern California)
Babesiosis	Parasite, *Babesia microti*	*Ixodes scapularis* (northeast of the US)

Abbreviation: US, United States.

BUG-BORNE DISEASE PREVENTION

Mosquito-Borne Disease

A number of arthropods, such as mosquitoes and ticks, can transmit diseases. Mosquito-vector diseases include West Nile virus, yellow fever virus, and dengue virus. West Nile virus, a flavivirus, has demonstrated a seasonally endemic epidemiology with geographic variation in the United States, especially in California, Arizona, and Colorado [7,61]. This disease typically presents between July and October, although cases have presented between April and December. The prevention of mosquito bites is the cornerstone of prevention. An athlete in an endemic area should wear an insect repellant such as deet (N,N-diethyl-m-toluamide), picaridin (KBR-3023), or oil of lemon eucalyptus (p-menthane-3,8 diol). Deet and permethin may be applied to the clothing [62]. If a sunscreen is used concomitantly, the insect repellant should be applied on top of this and removed at the end of the day. Long-sleeved shirts that are tucked into long pants are also useful.

Tick-Borne Disease

Tick-borne diseases include rickettsial diseases, Lyme disease, babesiosis, tick-borne relapsing fever, and occasionally, tularemia and Q fever (Table 5).

Table 5
Suggested resources for preventing infections

Topic	Web site
Vaccines licensed for immunization and distribution in the United States	www.fda.gov/cber/vaccine/licvacc.htm
	http://www.vaccineinformation.org/
How to store and handle vaccines	www.cdc.gov/nip/menus/ vaccines.htm#Storage
Adult immunization schedule	http://www.cdc.gov/nip/recs/ adult-schedule.htm
Travel information	www.cdc.gov/travel
	www.who.int/ith
Children and adolescents immunization schedule	http://www.cdc.gov/nip/recs/ child-schedule.htm
HIV position statements	http://www.fims.org/ (International Federation of Sports Medicine)
	http://www.casm-acms.org/forms/ statements/HIVEng.pdf (Canadian Academy of Sport Medicine)
	http://www.amssm.org/hiv.html (American Medical Society for Sports Medicine and the American Orthopaedic Society for Sports Medicine)
Morbidity and Mortality Weekly Reports	www.cdc.gov/mmwr
Primer for physicians for preventing food-borne illnesses	http://www.cdc.gov/mmwr/preview/ mmwrhtml/rr5002a1.htm

Web sites accessed November 3, 2006.

Certain athletes who participate in rural outdoor activities are more susceptible to tick bites. These sports include cross-country running, training in multiple sports in rural areas, and recreational outdoor sports such as fishing and hiking. Children are more at risk to tick bites.

Three more common rickettsial illnesses are Rocky Mountain spotted fever, human monocytotropic ehrlichiosis, and human granulocytotropic anaplasmosis [60]. The infectious organisms responsible for these illnesses maintain their lifecycles in mammals and ticks. Their prevalence reflects the geographic locations and the seasonality of the tick abundance. Their season is usually from April to September, but they can present throughout the year. Newer rickettsial diseases are emerging. These potentially lethal diseases are difficult to diagnose because they often mimic viral syndromes. As many as 60% to 75% of patients are initially misdiagnosed [63,64].

With Rocky Mountain spotted fever, more than 50% of cases are reported in the five states of North Carolina, South Carolina, Tennessee, Oklahoma, and Arkansas [65]. The presentation most often manifests as a sudden febrile illness with headache, myalgia, and a maculopapular rash that spreads in a centripetal pattern. *Rickettsia rickettsii* has a predilection for endothelial cells and can cause a diffuse vasculitis and an untreated mortality of 10%. The diagnosis is based on clinical presentation, with epidemiologic, geographic, and seasonal considerations. Laboratory testing may be supportive with thrombocytopenia and mild liver enzyme elevation. Serologic testing is supportive only on a delayed basis with acute and convalescent titers. Human monocytotropic ehrlichiosis and human granulocytotropic anaplasmosis can also present with acute headache, fever, and myalgia. Laboratory evaluation often demonstrates leukopenia, thrombocytopenia, and transaminase elevation.

Common tick-borne illnesses that have been reported in the northeast United States are Lyme disease and babesiosis, which are transmitted by the tick *Ixodes scapularis* [66]. Babesiosis can cause a febrile illness and possibly life-threatening anemia and thrombocytopenia. Lyme disease is a rickettsial disease caused by *Borrelia burgdorferi*. As such, concurrent disease may be caused by the same tick bite (see Table 4).

Tick-bite prevention

There are no proven vaccines for these tick-borne illnesses, but all are preventable by careful vigilance and protection. The key to prevention is to understand the regional epidemiology and seasonality of the diseases. Vaccination for Lyme disease (LYMErix) was originally approved; however, the manufacturer took the vaccine off the market due to declining sales. There was a 49% efficacy after two doses and a 76% efficacy after three doses [67]; however, the protection diminished after 2 years.

Ticks thrive in a wooded environment and at the edge of woods with surrounding high vegetation. Ticks are uncommon in well-mowed lawns. Relative tick-free zones can be created by placing wood chips or gravel around recreational areas to separate the woods [68]. Other landscape management tips include removing clippings and leaves, keeping stone walls clean of leaves, and restricting the use of groundcover, such as pachysandra, where pets and children may play. Widening woodland trails andkeeping in the center of the trail while walking may be helpful. When traveling in wooded areas, light-colored clothing is helpful to identify the tick. Long pants tucked into tightly woven socks and closed shoes minimize exposure. Deet at 10% to 25% should be applied to the skin. Permethrin may be applied only to the clothing. Clothes should be removed and cleaned and dried after exposure. The clothes dryer is effective in killing ticks. One should carefully check for ticks in the nymphal phase that may be the size of a pin head. Careful inspection should be done of the hair, ears, axilla, belly button, and legs. Children and pets should also be checked. It is also important to monitor pets that may travel in the woods and return indoors.

The technique of tick removal is critical. Tweezers with fine tips should be used close to the skin and pulled directly away. Squeezing the body may allow contamination of the disease into the host [69]. Lyme disease is not contracted until at least 24 hours of tick adherence [70]; however, ehrlichiosis may transmit in less than 24 hours. Preventive antibiotics are generally not indicated because less than 5% of bites are Lyme infected, especially with a flat tick. After a high-risk exposure (when the tick has been engaged for more than 24 hours and is engorged), a single dose of 200 mg of doxycycline is believed to be effective [71].

HYGIENE PRECAUTIONS AND INFECTION CONTROL
Personal Hygiene
Most infectious diseases are spread from contact with the microorganism directly or indirectly from the infected individual. Athletes frequently interact with teammates, coaches, athletic trainers, and physicians and share equipment, water bottles, towels, and supplies. This interaction is particularly a concern, with the recent outbreaks of methicillin-resistent *Staphylococcus aureus* (MRSA) infections among sports teams [72,73]. Three categories of potential risk factors for spreading infection have been suggested: "sharing" (sharing soap/towels/water bottles with teammates), "skin injury" (cuts, abrasions), and "close contact" (locker adjacent to infected teammate, living on-campus) [74].

Good personal hygiene can help reduce colonization of bacteria. Bacterial counts can range from 5000 to 5 million colony-forming units per square centimeter on the hands [75]. Universal body fluid precautions–for example, using disposable gloves when examining the oral cavity or wounds and frequent hand washing–can reduce the risk of infection. MRSA is transmitted from an infected patient to the gloves of a health care worker in approximately 17% (9%–25%). Physicians, in particular, have a low compliance for using gloves and washing their hands [76]. Proper surgical hand washing is recommended to be 15 to 30 seconds with soap, a 30-second rinse with water, followed by complete drying with a towel. The use of rinses and gels with concentrations of 50% to 95% alcohol take 15 seconds to use and are effective at killing organisms [75]. The use of chlorhexidine soap has been useful for reducing MRSA infections.

Viruses and bacteria can exist on equipment. MRSA was found in the taping gel and whirlpool in the training facilities of a professional football team [72]. Using diluted bleach (1 part bleach in 9 parts water) to cleanse training areas and equipment is recommended [8]. Routine cleaning schedules for shared equipment should be established and recorded.

For upper respiratory tract infections, isolation of those who have had close contact with someone who has a confirmed or suspected infection, especially those who have active symptoms such as persistent fever and cough, is an effective and practical method of avoiding contact [8].

Any athlete who has a scratch, abrasion, or laceration or who has potentially infectious skin lesions such as vesicular or weeping skin lesions should be removed from play until the area can be securely covered with occlusive bandages or dressings to prevent leakage of blood or serous fluid [77]. Uniforms with fresh blood should be removed and replaced immediately after stopping any bleeding. Bleach diluted with tap water in a 1:10 ratio can be used to wash equipment that has had contact with blood or body fluid. Body substance precautions should be taken by health care professionals at all times when treating open wounds.

Prevention of Methicillin-Resistant Staphylococcus Aureus

One type of bacteria that has become more common in the hospital and a community-acquired infection is MRSA. Although contact sports such as wrestling and football have been commonly associated with MRSA spread, this infection has also been discovered in minimal-contact sports such as fencing [78]. Three factors are associated with MRSA spread in sports. First, even with sports that have minimal contact, there are often abrasions and chaffing from clothing and hot environments. Second, equipment is often shared and there is potential for transmission of bacteria. Third, many sports have sufficient skin-to-skin contact to transmit organisms. Subsequently, health care providers should strongly encourage good overall and hand hygiene in addition to covering all wounds and limiting shared equipment. It is crucial to have an ample supply of soap and water and alcohol-based hand cleansers. Athletes, staff, and coaches should be educated in proper first aid for wounds, in recognition of wounds that are potentially infected, and in seeking medical attention for lesions that have concerning signs, especially large pustules or boils.

Prevention of Fungal Rashes

Athlete's foot, tinea pedis, is a common ailment not only during the hot summer months but also during the winter months with indoor sports. A number of prevention items include washing feet daily; drying between the toes; wearing cotton, nonsynthetic socks; wearing bathing shoes in public showers; and wearing sandals in warmer weather. Jock itch, tinea cruris, is best prevented by showering immediately after athletic endeavors and wearing cotton briefs. A good talc powder may be used for prevention of athlete's foot and jock itch. Ring worm, tinea corporis, is best prevented by avoiding contact. Contact athletes such as wrestlers should not participate until any lesions have cleared or can be safely and effectively covered.

SEXUALLY TRANSMITTED DISEASE PREVENTION

Athletes may manifest risk-taking behavior and subsequently be at increased risk for STDs [2]. The preparticipation examination affords the opportunity for the clinician to address these concerns. The CDC has emphasized the five intervention strategies [79], which include education on sexual behavior, identification of asymptomatic individuals, diagnosis and treatment of infected individuals, counseling of sexual partners of persons who have an STD, and pre-exposure vaccination when applicable. Individuals at risk should be questioned about partners regarding number and same or opposite sex. Information about the type of sexual activity, the use of protection, and history of previous STDs should also be identified.

Preventive measures for an STD include abstinence if an individual or partner is actively infected and undergoing treatment. Pre-exposure prophylaxis is relevant in several situations. Hepatitis B vaccine is recommended in all individuals potentially exposed to STDs. Hepatitis A vaccine is recommended for all men who have sex with men or users of illicit drugs (injectable and non-injectable). For girls and women aged 9 to 26 years, the new quadrivalent vaccine for HPV types 6, 11,16, and 18 is recommended due to the higher associated risk of cervical cancer.

Most condoms are made of latex and are quite effective in STD prevention. In one study of partners of HIV-infected individuals, partners were 80% less likely to seroconvert than those who did not use condoms [80]. The male condom can also reduce the transmission of gonorrhea, chlamydiosis, and trichomiasis [81]. There may be some added protection against herpes simplex virus 2 and a 70% reduction of HPV transmission [82,83]. When an individual is allergic to latex, certain polyurethane condoms are likely just as effective, although they may break more readily. Conversely, natural-membrane condoms such as lambskin are too porous to be used for STD prevention. Only water-based lubricants should be used with latex condoms because oil bases will weaken the latex. The female condom is a double-ringed polyurethane sheath that is used vaginally and during anal receptive intercourse that is effective in limited trials in preventing HIV/STDs [84,85]. Spermicides and nonbarrier contraception have no role in STD prevention.

Finally, providers should encourage patients who have STDs to notify their partners. Often, this notification is pursued by the public health department. In the event of exposure to HIV by sexual exposure or needle stick, HIV prophylaxis is often undertaken and should be immediate. Prophylactic treatment usually involves the hospital infectious disease division to determine the best combination therapy.

SUMMARY

Education is paramount in public health and in the prevention of infectious diseases. Athletes are a high-risk population often due to their increased exposure to different people and environments and, sometimes, their outgoing lifestyle behaviors. Primary prevention can be promoted through accurate immunizations; appropriate, planned health maintenance; good hygiene practices; and behavior modification to minimize high-risk activities. Secondary prevention can be achieved through vigilant surveillance for reportable illnesses, proper education and containment for reducing spread if an illness occurs, and timely prophylaxis with medications and immunizations in certain cases.

References

[1] Roberts JA, Wilson JA, Clements GB. Virus infections and sports performance—a prospective study. Br J Sports Med 1988;22(4):161–2.
[2] Nattiv A, Puffer JC, Green GA. Lifestyles and health risks of collegiate athletes: a multi-center study. Clin J Sport Med 1997;7(4):262–72.
[3] Ehresmann KR, Hedberg CW, Grimm MB, et al. An outbreak of measles at an international sporting event with airborne transmission in a domed stadium. J Infect Dis 1995;171(3):679–83.
[4] Tarrant M, Challis EB. Influenza vaccination for athletes? CMAJ 1988;139(4):282.

[5] Plasencia A, Segura A, Farres J, et al. Pneumococcal vaccine for Olympic athletes and visitors to Spain. Barcelona Olympic Organizing Committee. N Engl J Med 1992;327(6): 437.

[6] Brennan RJ, Keim ME, Sharp TW, et al. Medical and public health services at the 1996 Atlanta Olympic Games: an overview. Med J Aust 1997;167(11–12):595–8.

[7] Jajosky RA, Hall PA, Adams DA, et al. Summary of notifiable diseases—United States, 2004. MMWR Morb Mortal Wkly Rep 2006;53(53):1–79.

[8] So RC, Ko J, Yuan YW, et al. Severe acute respiratory syndrome and sport: facts and fallacies. Sports Med 2004;34(15):1023–33.

[9] Smith NM, Bresee JS, Shay DK, et al. Prevention and control of influenza: recommendations of the Advisory Committee on Immunization Practices (ACIP). MMWR Recomm Rep 2006;55(RR-10):1–42.

[10] Centers for Disease Control and Prevention. Basic information about SARS. Available at: http://www.cdc.gov/ncidod/SARS/factsheet.htm. Accessed November 3, 2006.

[11] Pate RR, Trost SG, Levin S, et al. Sports participation and health-related behaviors among US youth. Arch Pediatr Adolesc Med 2000;154(9):904–11.

[12] Sklarek HM, Mantovani RP, Erens E, et al. AIDS in a bodybuilder using anabolic steroids. N Engl J Med 1984;311(26):1701.

[13] Scott MJ, Scott MJ Jr. HIV infection associated with injections of anabolic steroids. JAMA 1989;262(2):207–8.

[14] Kordi R, Wallace WA. Blood borne infections in sport: risks of transmission, methods of prevention, and recommendations for hepatitis B vaccination. Br J Sports Med 2004;38(6):678–84 [discussion: 678–84].

[15] Rich JD, Dickinson BP, Feller A, et al. The infectious complications of anabolic-androgenic steroid injection. Int J Sports Med 1999;20(8):563–6.

[16] American Academy of Pediatrics, et al. Active and passive immunization. In: Pickering LK, Baker CJ, Long SS, editors. Red book: 2006 report of the Committee of Infectious Diseases. 27th edition. Elk Grove Village (IL): American Academy of Pediatrics; 2006. p. 1–93.

[17] Ehresmann KR, White KE, Hedberg CW, et al. A statewide survey of immunization rates in Minnesota school age children: implications for targeted assessment and prevention strategies. Pediatr Infect Dis J 1998;17(8):711–6.

[18] Tallia AF, Ibsen KH, Howarth DF. Swanson's family practice review: a problem-oriented approach. 5th edition. Philadelphia: Elsevier Inc.; 2005:468.

[19] Cote TR, Sivertson D, Horan JM, et al. Evaluation of a two-dose measles, mumps, and rubella vaccination schedule in a cohort of college athletes. Public Health Rep 1993;108(4): 431–5.

[20] Mufson MA. Antibody response of pneumococcal vaccine: need for booster dosing? Int J Antimicrob Agents 2000;14(2):107–12.

[21] Brown LS Jr, Drotman DP, Chu A, et al. Bleeding injuries in professional football: estimating the risk for HIV transmission. Ann Intern Med 1995;122(4):273–4.

[22] Kashiwagi S, Hayashi J, Ikematsu H, et al. An outbreak of hepatitis B in members of a high school sumo wrestling club. JAMA 1982;248(2):213–4.

[23] Tobe K, Matsuura K, Ogura T, et al. Horizontal transmission of hepatitis B virus among players of an American football team. Arch Intern Med 2000;160(16):2541–5.

[24] Mast EE, Margolis HS, Fiore AE, et al. A comprehensive immunization strategy to eliminate transmission of hepatitis B virus infection in the United States: recommendations of the Advisory Committee on Immunization Practices (ACIP) part 1: immunization of infants, children, and adolescents. MMWR Recomm Rep 2005;54(RR-16):1–31.

[25] American Academy of Pediatrics, et al. Hepatitis B. In: Pickering LK, Baker CJ, Long SS, editors. Red book: 2006 report of the Committee of Infectious Diseases. 27th edition. Elk Grove Village (IL): American Academy of Pediatrics; 2006. p. 169–71.

[26] Gregory DS. Pertussis: a disease affecting all ages. Am Fam Physician 2006;74(3): 420–6.

[27] Wendelboe AM, Van Rie A, Salmaso S, et al. Duration of immunity against pertussis after natural infection or vaccination. Pediatr Infect Dis J 2005;24(Suppl 5):S58–61.

[28] Hopkins RS, Jajosky RA, Hall PA, et al. Summary of notifiable diseases—United States, 2003. MMWR Morb Mortal Wkly Rep 2005;52(54):1–85.

[29] Olin P, Rasmussen F, Gustafsson L, et al. Randomised controlled trial of two-component, three-component, and five-component acellular pertussis vaccines compared with whole-cell pertussis vaccine. Ad Hoc Group for the Study of Pertussis Vaccines. Lancet 1997;350(9091):1569–77.

[30] Jefferson T, Rudin M, DiPietrantonj C. Systematic review of the effects of pertussis vaccines in children. Vaccine 2003;21(17–18):2003–14.

[31] Broder KR, Cortese MM, Iskander JK, et al. Preventing tetanus, diphtheria, and pertussis among adolescents: use of tetanus toxoid, reduced diphtheria toxoid and acellular pertussis vaccines recommendations of the Advisory Committee on Immunization Practices (ACIP). MMWR Recomm Rep 2006;55(RR-3):1–34.

[32] American Academy of Pediatrics, et al. Pertussis. In: Pickering LK, Baker CJ, Long SS, editors. Red book: 2006 report of the Committee of Infectious Diseases. 27th edition. Elk Grove Village (IL): American Academy of Pediatrics; 2006. p. 472–86.

[33] Loeffelholz MJ, Thompson CJ, Long KS, et al. Comparison of PCR, culture, and direct fluorescent-antibody testing for detection of Bordetella pertussis. J Clin Microbiol 1999;37(9):2872–6.

[34] Tiwari T, Murphy TV, Moran J. Recommended antimicrobial agents for the treatment and postexposure prophylaxis of pertussis: 2005 CDC guidelines. MMWR Recomm Rep 2005;54(RR-14):1–16.

[35] Lyytikainen O, Hoffmann E, Timm H, et al. Influenza A outbreak among adolescents in a ski hostel. Eur J Clin Microbiol Infect Dis 1998;17(2):128–30.

[36] Wilde JA, McMillan JA, Serwint J, et al. Effectiveness of influenza vaccine in health care professionals: a randomized trial. JAMA 1999;281(10):908–13.

[37] Brokstad KA, Cox RJ, Olofsson J, et al. Parenteral influenza vaccination induces a rapid systemic and local immune response. J Infect Dis 1995;171(1):198–203.

[38] Belshe RB, Nichol KL, Black SB, et al. Safety, efficacy, and effectiveness of live, attenuated, cold-adapted influenza vaccine in an indicated population aged 5–49 years. Clin Infect Dis 2004;39(7):920–7.

[39] Nichol KL, Mendelman PM, Mallon KP, et al. Effectiveness of live, attenuated intranasal influenza virus vaccine in healthy, working adults: a randomized controlled trial. JAMA 1999;282(2):137–44.

[40] Ross DS, Swain R, Thomas J. Study indicates influenza vaccine beneficial for college athletes. W V Med J 2001;97(5):235.

[41] Matsumoto K, Ogawa N, Nerome K, et al. Safety and efficacy of the neuraminidase inhibitor zanamivir in treating influenza virus infection in adults: results from Japan. GG167 Group. Antivir Ther 1999;4(2):61–8.

[42] Cooper NJ, Sutton AJ, Abrams KR, et al. Effectiveness of neuraminidase inhibitors in treatment and prevention of influenza A and B: systematic review and meta-analyses of randomised controlled trials. BMJ 2003;326(7401):1235–43.

[43] Bright RA, Shay DK, Shu B, et al. Adamantane resistance among influenza A viruses isolated early during the 2005–2006 influenza season in the United States. JAMA 2006;295(8):891–4.

[44] Kaiser L, Wat C, Mills T, et al. Impact of oseltamivir treatment on influenza-related lower respiratory tract complications and hospitalizations. Arch Intern Med 2003;163(14):1667–72.

[45] Jefferson T, Demicheli V, Rivetti D, et al. Antivirals for influenza in healthy adults: systematic review. Lancet 2006;367(9507):303–13.

[46] Uhnoo I, Linde A, Pauksens K, et al. Treatment and prevention of influenza: Swedish recommendations. Scand J Infect Dis 2003;35(1):3–11.

[47] Gundlapalli AV, Rubin MA, Samore MH, et al. Influenza, winter Olympiad, 2002. Emerg Infect Dis 2006;12(1):144–6.
[48] Rodriguez WJ, Schwartz RH, Thorne MM. Evaluation of diagnostic tests for influenza in a pediatric practice. Pediatr Infect Dis J 2002;21(3):193–6.
[49] Uyeki TM. Influenza diagnosis and treatment in children: a review of studies on clinically useful tests and antiviral treatment for influenza. Pediatr Infect Dis J 2003;22(2):164–77.
[50] Bilukha OO, Rosenstein N. Prevention and control of meningococcal disease. Recommendations of the Advisory Committee on Immunization Practices (ACIP). MMWR Recomm Rep 2005;54(RR-7):1–21.
[51] Bruce MG, Rosenstein NE, Capparella JM, et al. Risk factors for meningococcal disease in college students. JAMA 2001;286(6):688–93.
[52] Control and prevention of meningococcal disease: recommendations of the Advisory Committee on Immunization Practices (ACIP). MMWR Recomm Rep 1997;46(RR-5):1–10.
[53] Trotter CL, Andrews NJ, Kaczmarski EB, et al. Effectiveness of meningococcal serogroup C conjugate vaccine 4 years after introduction. Lancet 2004;364(9431):365–7.
[54] Girgis N, Sultan Y, Frenck RW Jr, et al. Azithromycin compared with rifampin for eradication of nasopharyngeal colonization by Neisseria meningitidis. Pediatr Infect Dis J 1998;17(9): 816–9.
[55] Moscicki AB, Hills N, Shiboski S, et al. Risks for incident human papillomavirus infection and low-grade squamous intraepithelial lesion development in young females. JAMA 2001;285(23):2995–3002.
[56] Winer RL, Lee SK, Hughes JP, et al. Genital human papillomavirus infection: incidence and risk factors in a cohort of female university students. Am J Epidemiol 2003;157(3):218–26.
[57] Harper DM, Franco EL, Wheeler CM, et al. Sustained efficacy up to 4.5 years of a bivalent L1 virus-like particle vaccine against human papillomavirus types 16 and 18: follow-up from a randomised control trial. Lancet 2006;367(9518):1247–55.
[58] CDC. ACIP provisional recommendations for the use of quadrivalent HPV vaccine. Available at: http://www.cdc.gov/nip/recs/provisional_recs/hpv.pdf. Accessed November 9, 2006.
[59] American Academy of Pediatrics, et al. Human papillomaviruses. In: Pickering LK, Baker CJ, Long SS, editors. Red book: 2006 report of the Committee of Infectious Diseases. 27th edition. Elk Grove Village (IL): American Academy of Pediatrics; 2006. p. 473–6.
[60] Carpenter CF, Gandhi TK, Kong LK, et al. The incidence of ehrlichial and rickettsial infection in patients with unexplained fever and recent history of tick bite in central North Carolina. J Infect Dis 1999;180(3):900–3.
[61] O'Leary DR, Marfin AA, Montgomery SP, et al. The epidemic of West Nile virus in the United States, 2002. Vector Borne Zoonotic Dis 2004;4(1):61–70.
[62] Barnard DR, Xue RD. Laboratory evaluation of mosquito repellents against Aedes albopictus, Culex nigripalpus, and Ochlerotatus triseriatus (Diptera: Culicidae). J Med Entomol 2004;41(4):726–30.
[63] O'Reilly M, Paddock C, Elchos B, et al. Physician knowledge of the diagnosis and management of Rocky Mountain spotted fever: Mississippi, 2002. Ann N Y Acad Sci 2003;990: 295–301.
[64] Helmick CG, Bernard KW, D'Angelo LJ. Rocky Mountain spotted fever: clinical, laboratory, and epidemiological features of 262 cases. J Infect Dis 1984;150(4):480–8.
[65] Treadwell TA, Holman RC, Clarke MJ, et al. Rocky Mountain spotted fever in the United States, 1993-1996. Am J Trop Med Hyg 2000;63(1–2):21–6.
[66] Herwaldt BL, McGovern PC, Gerwel MP, et al. Endemic babesiosis in another eastern state: New Jersey. Emerg Infect Dis 2003;9(2):184–8.
[67] Steere AC, Sikand VK, Meurice F, et al. Vaccination against Lyme disease with recombinant Borrelia burgdorferi outer-surface lipoprotein A with adjuvant. Lyme Disease Vaccine Study Group. N Engl J Med 1998;339(4):209–15.
[68] Couch P, Johnson CE. Prevention of Lyme disease. Am J Hosp Pharm 1992;49(5):1164–73.

[69] des Vignes F, Piesman J, Heffernan R, et al. Effect of tick removal on transmission of *Borrelia burgdorferi* and *Ehrlichia phagocytophila* by *Ixodes scapularis* nymphs. J Infect Dis 2001;183(5):773–8.

[70] Falco RC, Fish D, Piesman J. Duration of tick bites in a Lyme disease-endemic area. Am J Epidemiol 1996;143(2):187–92.

[71] Nadelman RB, Nowakowski J, Fish D, et al. Prophylaxis with single-dose doxycycline for the prevention of Lyme disease after an *Ixodes scapularis* tick bite. N Engl J Med 2001;345(2): 79–84.

[72] Kazakova SV, Hageman JC, Matava M, et al. A clone of methicillin-resistant *Staphylococcus aureus* among professional football players. N Engl J Med 2005;352(5):468–75.

[73] Lindenmayer JM, Schoenfeld S, O'Grady R, et al. Methicillin-resistant *Staphylococcus aureus* in a high school wrestling team and the surrounding community. Arch Intern Med 1998;158(8):895–9.

[74] Nguyen DM, Mascola L, Brancoft E. Recurring methicillin-resistant *Staphylococcus aureus* infections in a football team. Emerg Infect Dis 2005;11(4):526–32.

[75] Gawande A. On washing hands. N Engl J Med 2004;350(13):1283–6.

[76] McBryde ES, Bradley LC, Whitby M, et al. An investigation of contact transmission of methicillin-resistant *Staphylococcus aureus*. J Hosp Infect 2004;58(2):104–8.

[77] Mast EE, Goodman RA, Bond WW, et al. Transmission of blood-borne pathogens during sports: risk and prevention. Ann Intern Med 1995;122(4):283–5.

[78] Gantz N, Harmon H, Handy J. Methicillin-resistant *Staphylococcus aureus* infections among competitive sports participants—Colorado, Indiana, Pennsylvania, and Los Angeles County, 2000–2003. MMWR Morb Mortal Wkly Rep 2003;52(33):793–5.

[79] Workowski KA, Berman SM. Sexually transmitted diseases treatment guidelines, 2006. MMWR Recomm Rep 2006;55(RR-11):1–94.

[80] Holmes KK, Levine R, Weaver M. Effectiveness of condoms in preventing sexually transmitted infections. Bull World Health Organ 2004;82(6):454–61.

[81] Wingood GM, DiClemente RJ, Mikhail I, et al. A randomized controlled trial to reduce HIV transmission risk behaviors and sexually transmitted diseases among women living with HIV: the WiLLOW Program. J Acquir Immune Defic Syndr 2004;37(Suppl 2):S58–67.

[82] Wald A, Langenberg AG, Link K, et al. Effect of condoms on reducing the transmission of herpes simplex virus type 2 from men to women. JAMA 2001;285(24):3100–6.

[83] Winer RL, Hughes JP, Feng Q, et al. Condom use and the risk of genital human papillomavirus infection in young women. N Engl J Med 2006;354(25):2645–54.

[84] French PP, Latka M, Gollub EL, et al. Use-effectiveness of the female versus male condom in preventing sexually transmitted disease in women. Sex Transm Dis 2003;30(5):433–9.

[85] Gross M, Buchbinder SP, Holte S, et al. Use of reality "female condoms" for anal sex by US men who have sex with men. HIVNET Vaccine Preparedness Study Protocol Team. Am J Public Health 1999;89(11):1739–41.

Clin Sports Med 26 (2007) 345–359

CLINICS IN SPORTS MEDICINE

ELSEVIER
SAUNDERS

Upper Respiratory Tract Infections in Athletes

Clifton L. Page, MD, Jason J. Diehl, MD*

Division of Sports Medicine, Department of Family Medicine, The Ohio State University Sports Medicine Center, 2050 Kenny Road, Columbus, OH 43221, USA

U pper respiratory tract infections (URTIs) represent the most common acute illnesses in the general population and account for the leading acute diagnoses in the outpatient setting [1]. Similarly, athletes are infected with these illnesses and require appropriate treatment, allowing them to participate safely and at their full potential. Groups of athletes are often at an elevated risk of transmission because they are confined to close quarters with teammates in the locker room, at practice, and during travel. Further evidence demonstrates a higher susceptibility to URTIs in athletes during and after high training loads, likely from a suppressed immune system [1]. Viruses account for most URTIs, but the sports medicine physician must be able to recognize bacterial infections and the potential complications that require specific therapy. Given the athlete's expectation to return to activity as soon as possible, the sports medicine physician should be able to accurately diagnose and aggressively treat these illnesses.

Management of URTIs in athletes spans a wide range of pathogens, clinical presentations, and treatment options. Participation and return-to-sport decisions are determined by the nature of the infection, the risk of transmission, and the demand placed on the athlete during practice and competition. Decisions should be made on a case-by-case basis using the best evidence-based medical care. Above all, any recommendations made should address the safety of the athlete and all participants involved. In this article, the authors discuss the common pathogens, diagnosis, treatment options, and return-to-play decisions for URTIs, with a focus on the common cold, sinusitis, pharyngitis, and infectious mononucleosis in the athlete.

VIRAL UPPER RESPIRATORY TRACT INFECTION (THE COMMON COLD)

The common cold is the most frequent acute illness in the United States and the leading cause of missed days from school or work [1]. A viral

*Corresponding author. E-mail address: jason.diehl@osumc.edu (J.J. Diehl).

0278-5919/07/$ – see front matter
doi:10.1016/j.csm.2007.04.001

URTI is a benign self-limiting syndrome typically lasting 5 to 14 days, manifested by rhinorrhea, cough, and fever and caused by multiple families of viruses. The pathogens most frequently associated with common cold symptoms are rhinoviruses (10%–40% of cases), coronaviruses (20%), and respiratory syncytial virus (10%) [2]. Influenza viruses, parainfluenza viruses, and adenoviruses also cause common cold symptoms, but to a lesser degree [2].

Direct contact, small-particle aerosols, and large-particle aerosols can spread common cold viruses. Person-to-person contact depends on the amount of time people spend together and the amount of virus shed by the infected donor [3]. In relatively closed communities, secondary attack rates can range from 25% to 70% [4]. Hand-to-hand contact is an important factor in the transmission of disease. The most efficient means of viral transmission is the spread of infectious mucoid secretions to the fingers and hands and subsequently to the nose or eyes of a susceptible person [5]. Some viruses can be viable on the human skin for at least 2 hours, and one study found that certain viruses could be recovered from 40% to 90% of hands of persons who have colds [5]. This ease of transmission demonstrates the need to encourage proper hand washing in the athletic population as an important preventive measure to reduce the number of illnesses and time away from sport.

The common cold can have more serious complications. Acute bacterial sinusitis develops in about 2.5% of adult patients after a viral URTI [6]. Infections can also be complicated by lower respiratory tract disease, such as pneumonia, and have been linked to up to 40% of acute asthma attacks in adults [7]. It is important for the sports medicine physician to readily identify the common symptoms of, properly diagnose, and effectively manage viral URTIs to reduce the more serious complications from the illness.

Diagnosis

Viral URTIs can be difficult to distinguish from less common bacterial cases solely based on clinical examination. Findings on physical examination are few in light of the subjective discomfort of the patient, and the symptoms may vary from patient to patient with the same illness. The incubation period for most common cold viruses is 24 to 72 hours [8]. Colds usually persist for 3 to 7 days in the normal host; however, 25% of colds may last as long as 2 weeks [2]. Risk factors that increase severity of disease include young age, low birth weight, prematurity, chronic disease, immunodeficiency disorders, malnutrition, and crowding [8].

Antiviral therapy is not available for most viruses that cause viral URTIs. Therefore, despite being the standard of confirmation, viral cultures are rarely indicated for uncomplicated URTIs in the outpatient setting [2]. Patients who have viral URTIs can have an increased white blood cell count associated with a left shift. Some viral infections can precipitate atypical lympocytes, lymphocytosis, or lymphopenia; however, a complete blood count is not helpful in distinguishing disease or in directing therapy in uncomplicated URTI in the outpatient setting [2].

Treatment and Return to Play

There is no evidence that antibiotics have a clinically important effect on colds uncomplicated by secondary infection. Symptomatic therapy remains the foundation of common cold treatment. A number of agents have been studied and have demonstrated varying effects on the course of illness (Table 1) [9–14].

Table 1
Treatment of upper respiratory infection

Treatment	Benefit	Data	Level of evidence [reference]
Antibiotics	Not likely beneficial		A[a] [9]
Decongestants	May be beneficial	Compared with placebo, a single dose of an oral or topical decongestant produced a significant 13% reduction in subjective symptoms There was no benefit from repeated use over several days There are limited data to support its use in children	A[a] [27]
Antihistamine	May be beneficial	Reduced the symptoms of runny nose and sneezing for the first 2 d of colds	A[a] [10]
Vitamin C	Unknown effectiveness	1 g daily or more produces about 15% fewer symptomatic days per episode	B[b] [11]
Zinc	Unknown effectiveness	May reduce duration of cold symptoms at 7 d compared with placebo Two randomized controlled trials found that zinc intranasal gel reduced the mean duration of cold symptoms compared with placebo	B[b] [12]
Echinacea	Unknown effectiveness	Some preparations of Echinacea may be better than placebo for cold treatment	B[b] [13]
Steam	Unknown effectiveness	Conflicting evidence of the efficacy of steam inhalation at 40°–47°C in the reduction of cold symptoms	B[b] [14]

[a]Level A is consistent, good-quality patient-oriented evidence (SORT evidence rating system).
[b]Level B is inconsistent or limited-quality patient-oriented evidence (SORT evidence rating system).

According to the American College of Sports Medicine, when an athlete has common cold symptoms without fever or general body aches and pains, intensive exercise training may be safely resumed a few days after the resolution of symptoms; mild-to-moderate exercise does not appear to be harmful for individuals who have common cold symptoms [15]. In settings with appropriate supervision, athletes who have viral URTIs and no fevers, myalgias, or symptoms below the neck are safe to continue their previous level of activity with no restrictions. Return-to-play decisions should be made on a case-by-case basis and should focus on minimizing the risk of further harm.

ACUTE SINUSITIS

Sinusitis is one of the most common illnesses diagnosed in the United States, affecting about 16% of the adult population annually [16]. Sinusitis is defined as inflammation of one or more of the paranasal sinuses and is categorized as acute (<4 weeks), subacute (4–8 weeks), and chronic (>8 weeks) [17]. The cause of sinusitis can be viral or bacterial (Table 2). Viral infection is the most common cause of acute sinusitis, and usually resolves in 7 to 10 days. Acute bacterial sinusitis is also usually a self-limiting disease, with 75% of cases resolving without treatment after 1 month [17]. When left untreated, however, bacterial sinusitis may not spontaneously resolve and can have severe complications including intracranial and orbital infections.

Diagnosis

The diagnosis of sinusitis is based on a combination of clinical history and physical examination findings. Imaging studies and laboratory tests can assist in the diagnosis of chronic or complicated cases. Symptoms of acute sinusitis include nasal congestion, purulent nasal discharge, maxillary tooth discomfort, headaches, fever, and facial pain or pressure that is worse when leaning forward [18]. It is unfortunate that the history is not sensitive or specific for

Table 2
Pathogens of acute sinusitis

Viral		Bacterial community-acquired[a]	
	Rhinovirus		Streptococcus pneumoniae
	Parainfluenza virus		Haemophilus influenza
	Influenza virus		Moraxella catarrhalis
	Corona virus		Other streptococcal species
	Respiratory syncytial virus		Staphylococcus aureus
	Adenovirus		Anaerobic bacteria

[a]The most common organisms are Streptococcus pneumoniae and Haemophilus influenza. These pathogens are responsible for 35% of cases in adults. In children, S pneumoniae and H influenza are responsible for 41% and 29% of cases, respectively. Moraxella catarrhalis accounts for 26% of cases in children and 2% in adults.

From Evans A, Niederman J. Epstein-Barr virus. In: Evans A, editor. Viral infections of human epidemiology and control. New York: Plenum Publishing; 1989. p. 265; with permission.

distinguishing between viral and bacterial infections [19]. Although the symptoms of sinusitis are nonspecific, a history of persistent purulent rhinorrhea and facial pain appear to have some correlation with increased likelihood of bacterial disease [20].

Physical examination including palpation of the sinuses, transillumination, and visualization of the nares does not assist in differentiating bacterial from viral sinusitis. Frequently, sinusitis presents with facial tenderness over the affected sinus cavity. Transillumination can be reported as opaque (no transmission), dull (reduced transmission) or normal, but the sensitivity and specificity of this technique is poor [21]. One prospective study found that abnormal transillumination combined with purulent nasal discharge and history of maxillary pain, poor response to decongestants, and colored rhinorrea was the best predictor of acute bacterial sinusitis [19].

Sinus aspirate culture is the "gold standard" for making microbial diagnosis, but it is not done routinely in clinical practice. Sinus aspiration should be considered when there is suspicion of intracranial extension of the infection or other serious complication.

Imaging studies are not usually indicated for noncomplicated cases of bacterial sinusitis but can provide confirmatory evidence when clinical disease persists despite optimal medical therapy. CT scanning is usually the procedure of choice and provides better sensitivity than plain radiographs (88% versus 59%) [22]. It is unfortunate that neither test can distinguish bacterial from viral infection, and CT scan is limited by the fact it can be frequently abnormal in patients who have the common cold. In one study, 27 of 31 adults who had a viral cold had abnormal CT of the sinuses, including occlusion and abnormalities in the sinus cavities [23]. In addition, MRI can be used to detect intracranial spread of infection, distinguish inflammatory disease and malignant tumor, and evaluate for fungal disease; however, MRI is not as good as CT scan in diagnosing acute sinusitis [23].

Treatment and Return to Play

Symptomatic treatment is the mainstay for the treatment of viral sinusitis, and antibiotics are generally not beneficial. Conversely, antibiotics are beneficial in the medical treatment for acute bacterial sinusitis. In patients who have an acute sinus infection, antibiotics are recommended when symptoms have not improved after 10 days, for severe illness, or when symptoms have worsened over 5 to 7 days [24]. The appropriate choice of antibiotic should be based on the most likely bacterial pathogen and clinical history. Current literature supports amoxicillin as the initial antibiotic choice in children and adults who have uncomplicated bacterial sinusitis [25,26]. A 10- to 14-day course of antibiotics is typically successful for the treatment of acute bacterial sinusitis [25].

Symptomatic treatments including antihistamines, decongestants, and nasal steroids may be beneficial in the treatment of viral and bacterial sinusitis. Despite being used to treat symptoms, antihistamines have not proved to be beneficial and were not recommended in recent guidelines for the diagnosis and management of sinusitis in children [25]. Decongestants decrease nasal resistance and may be beneficial in the management of acute sinusitis; however, there has been relatively little systematic study of decongestants in patients who have sinusitis [27]. Intranasal steroids are also commonly used for the treatment of sinusitis, but until there is more evidence on the use of intranasal steroids in acute bacterial sinusitis, their use is not recommended [26].

Because acute viral sinusitis is a self-limiting illness and symptoms usually resolve in 7 to 10 days, exercise may be permitted with appropriate symptomatic care, particularly if the symptoms remain from the neck up (nasal congestion, facial pain, headaches, and so forth). When the athlete presents with more severe symptoms, however, including fevers or myalgias, vigorous exercise should be avoided to prevent dehydration and worsening of symptoms. Further, if the athlete's symptoms worsen after 5 to 7 days or persist longer than 10 days, appropriate antibiotic treatment should be initiated and participation allowed as tolerated.

ACUTE PHARYNGITIS (SORE THROAT)

Acute pharyngitis accounts for 19 million clinic visits annually and relates to about 2% of all ambulatory visits in the United States [28]. Acute pharyngitis can be caused by viral and bacterial pathogens. Viral causes account for approximately 50% of acute pharyngitis infections and can cause pharyngitis indistinguishable from bacterial pharyngitis [29]. These viral agents include influenza virus, parainfluenza virus, coronavirus, rhinovirus, adenovirus, enterovirus, herpes simplex virus, Epstein-Barr virus (EBV), and HIV. Because of the potential complications, the major treatable pathogen is group A streptococcus (GAS), but this accounts for only about 10% of adult cases [29]. Other bacterial pathogens include group C and group G streptococcus, mixed anaerobes, *Neisseria gonorrhoea*, *Corynebacterium diptheriae*, and several chlamydial species. Even though the differential diagnosis of acute pharyngitis in adults includes several viral and bacterial pathogens, the risk of rheumatic fever, acute glomerulonephritis, and supportive complications can be minimized by efficient and accurate diagnosis and treatment of GAS pharyngitis.

Diagnosis

For appropriate treatment, it is important to differentiate viral causes from bacterial causes, especially GAS. Viral pharyngitis has some associated clinical findings including pharyngeal swelling, erythema, and exudates. Furthermore, the presence of cough is more suggestive of a viral etiology. Primary herpes simplex virus infection may also be associated with palatal vesicles or shallow ulcers. Bacterial pharyngitis can be difficult to distinguish from viral pharyngitis clinically; however, a constellation of symptoms has been used to suggest GAS infection, including erythema, swelling, exudates of the tonsils or pharynx, fever (38.3°C/100.9°F or higher), tender anterior cervical lymph nodes, and absence of conjunctivitis, cough, or rhinorrhea [30]. A scarlet rash may be seen with GAS infections, particularly in patients younger than 18 years [31]. It appears as tiny papules over the chest and abdomen, often described as sandpaper-like. The rash spreads and becomes more erythematous in the groin and armpits, usually resolving within 2 to 5 days.

Laboratory evaluation can assist the clinician in identifying GAS infection. Throat cultures remain the gold standard for diagnosing GAS pharyngitis and may isolate other pathogens. With proper technique, the sensitivity for throat cultures approaches 90% and the specificity ranges from 95% to 99% [32]. False positive results can be linked to a 1% to 5% carrier rate for the organism [33]. Cultures take 24 to 48 hours to grow and cannot immediately be used for clinical decisions on whether to start antibiotics. Therefore, the rapid streptococcal antigen test (RSAT) has emerged as the first test of choice in the management of acute pharyngitis. Studies show a sensitivity of 80% to 90% and a specificity of 90% to 100% [28]. Although less sensitive than throat cultures, the RSAT provides results in minutes and can assist in same-day management.

Treatment and Return to Play

Symptomatic care alone is appropriate for most acute pharyngitis cases. The major exception is GAS pharyngitis, which requires appropriate antibiotic treatment to prevent potential complications, to minimize secondary spread, and to shorten the course of the illness (Table 3) [34,35]. In athletes who are sexually active, the clinician may need to consider gonococcal infections as a cause of acute pharyngitis. Gonococcal infections are easily treatable with proper antibiotics.

It has been found that nonsteroidal anti-inflammatory drugs (NSAIDs) reduced sore throat symptoms at 24 hours or less and at 2 to 5 days compared with placebo [36]. Caution must be advised when prescribing NSAIDs, however, because they are associated with gastrointestinal and renal adverse effects. Studies in children and adolescents who had moderate to severe sore throat but without group A beta hemolytic GAS infection have shown that oral dexamethasone reduced time to initial pain relief and duration of throat pain compared with placebo. Adding corticosteroids to antibiotics, however, did not significantly reduce pain duration in children and adolescents who had group A beta hemolytic GAS infection [37].

In athletes who have suspected or confirmed acute bacterial pharyngitis, it is important to remember that they are considered contagious until they have been on antibiotic therapy for 24 hours, and it is recommended that they not participate until this time has passed [38]. Treated appropriately, individuals should see improvement in acute symptoms within 24 hours and may progress to activity as tolerated. Under close supervision, removal from competition is often unnecessary if the athlete has no fevers or systemic symptoms (Table 4) [39–43].

Table 3
Antibiotic therapy for acute bacterial sinusitis

Antibiotic	Treatment	Adult dosage	Pediatric dosage	Data	Level of evidence
First-line antibiotics					
Amoxicillin	10 d	500 mg bid	45 mg/kg bid	Increased recovery rates compared with placebo at 2 wk 7–10 d of amoxicillin significantly increased complete symptom resolution compared with placebo	A[a] [34,35]
	If no response after 72 h, re-evaluate and consider alternative antibiotics				
Doxycycline		100 mg bid	2.2 mg/kg bid	Increased recovery rates compared with placebo at 2 wk	A[a] [34]
Trimethoprim-sulfamethoxazole		160/800 mg bid	40/200 mg/kg bid		
Alternative antibiotics					
Amoxicillin/ clavulanate		500–875 mg bid	22.5–45 mg/kg bid		
Cefpodoxime		200–400 mg bid	5 mg/kg bid		
Cefuroxime		250–500 mg bid	7.5 mg/kg bid		
Cefixime		400 mg qd	8 mg/kg qd		
Azithromycin		250 mg qd	5 mg/kg qd		
Clarithromycin		500 mg bid	7.5 mg/kg bid		
Levofloxacin		500 mg bid			

Blank entry, not recommended.
[a]Level A is consistent, good-quality patient-oriented evidence (SORT evidence rating system).

INFECTIOUS MONONUCLEOSIS

Infectious mononucleosis (mono) is a common illness in young adults, including the athletic population. Mono occurs in 3% of the college population and is characterized by the triad of fever, tonsillar pharyngitis, and lymphadenopathy [44]. It has long been accepted that EBV is the infectious pathogen of mono. EBV is a widely disseminated herpesvirus that is spread by intimate contact between susceptible hosts and asymptomatic EBV shedders. Often called the "kissing disease," EBV primarily spreads by way of the passage of saliva. The virus can persist in the oropharynx of patients who have a history of mono for up to 18 months after clinical recovery. Often, the illness can go undiagnosed if the symptoms are mild, but adolescents and young adults develop symptoms with higher frequency, ranging from 50% to 70% [45].

Although mono is generally a benign illness, splenic rupture is a known serious complication of mono, with an estimated occurrence of 1 to 2 cases per 1000 [46]. Almost all of the reported cases have occurred in male patients [45]. On occasion, splenic rupture is the first presenting symptom of mono, and it is spontaneous in over half of reported cases, with no history of impact or inciting injury [12]. Vital to the return-to-play decision, splenic rupture occurs primarily between the fourth and 21st day of symptomatic illness [45]. Despite being potentially life threatening, fatality from splenic rupture is rare.

Diagnosis

Classic mono presents with moderate to high fever, pharyngitis, and lymphadenopathy. One study of over 500 patients demonstrated that lymphadenopathy occurred in 100%, fever occurred in 98%, and pharyngitis occurred in 85% of documented cases [44]. Posterior cervical lymph nodes are characteristically more involved than anterior chains in mono, and these nodes may be large and moderately tender [44]. Lymphadenopathy peaks in the first week and gradually resolves over 2 to 3 weeks. The pharyngitis of mono is commonly described as exudative that may appear white, gray-green, or display necrotic features. Other findings include severe fatigue and splenomegaly. In a study of 631 Division I collegiate athletes, mean splenic size was 10.65 cm in length and 5.16 cm wide. Seven percent of the athletes' baseline spleen size met the current criteria for splenomegaly [47]. In this population, a single ultrasound evaluation of spleen size is of limited value, and clinical judgment may be more useful. Splenomegaly associated with mono occurs in 50% to 60% of patients and usually recedes by the third week of illness [48].

Laboratory information can be important in the confirmation of the diagnosis of mono. A peripheral blood smear commonly shows a white blood cell count of 12,000/mm^3 to 18,000/mm^3 and a differential showing 60% to 70% lymphocytes, with more than 10% of these being atypical [49]. In contrast to the finding of atypical lympocytes, heterophile antibodies are sensitive and specific for mono (85% and 100%, respectively) [49]. Heterophile antibodies

Table 4
Antibiotic therapy for acute pharyngitis

Drug/dosage	Advantages	Disadvantages	Data/Level of evidence [reference]
Penicillin V potassium	Inexpensive		First drug of choice; reduces streptococcal complications compared with placebo/A[a] [39]
<23 kg: 250 mg bid or tid × 10 d	Narrow spectrum of antibacterial activity		
>23 kg: 500 mg bid or tid × 10 d or 250 mg bid or tid	Low side effect profile Twice-daily dosing		
Penicillin G benzathine	Ensures compliance	Pain at injection site	
<27 kg: 600,000 U intramuscularly × 1 dose		Possible allergic reaction Cannot discontinue drug exposure if allergy develops	
>27 kg: 1.2 million U intramuscularly × 1 dose			
Erythromycin	Resistance is uncommon in the United States	Gastrointestinal upset	Drug of choice in penicillin-allergic patients
Estolate	No difference in cure rate with all forms		Equally as effective as penicillin in preventing all complications of group A streptococcus/B[b] [40]
20–30 mg/kg divided bid-qid × 10 d			
Ethyl succinate or sterate			
<41 kg: 40 mg/kg/d divided bid-qid × 10 d			
>41 kg: 400 mg qid × 10 d			

Cephalexin Pediatric: 25–50 mg/kg/d divided bid × 10 d Adults: 500 mg bid × 10 d	Twice-daily dosing	Broader spectrum	Equal cure rate versus oral penicillin/ B[b] [41]
Clindamycin Pediatric: 20 mg/kg/d divided tid × 10 d Adults: 450 mg/d divided tid × 10 d	Unaffected by beta lactamase Narrow spectrum Eliminates carrier status	Expensive Potential to develop Stevens-Johnson syndrome Pseudomembranous colitis may occur up to several weeks after stopping therapy	C[c] [42]

Blank entry, not recommended.
[a] Level A is consistent, good-quality patient-oriented evidence (SORT evidence rating system).
[b] Level B is inconsistent or limited-quality patient-oriented evidence (SORT evidence rating system).
[c] Level C recommendation is based on consensus, usual practice, opinion, disease-oriented evidence, or case series for studies of diagnosis, treatment, prevention, or screening.

appear within 1 week of the onset of clinical symptoms, peak in weeks 2 to 5, and may persist at low levels for up to 12 months. Measurements of EBV-specific antibodies are often obtained in lieu of the heterophile antibodies in athletes because they can determine the acuity of the illness.

Treatment and Return to Play

The mainstay of treatment for patients who have mono is supportive care. The treatment and return-to-play decision making is geared toward reducing the probability of splenic rupture. Acetaminophen or NSAIDs are recommended for the treatment of fever, pharyngitis, and malaise. It is important to stress adequate fluid and nutrition intake; adequate rest is necessary, but strict bed rest is not warranted. Corticosteroid and antiviral therapies have been studied in the treatment of mono. In a multicenter placebo-controlled trial of 94 patients who had acute mono, the combination of acyclovir and prednisolone reduced oropharygeal shedding of the virus but did not affect the duration of symptoms or lead to earlier return to school or work [50]. Further, a meta-analysis of five randomized controlled trials of acyclovir in the treatment of acute mono failed to show a clinical benefit compared with placebo [51].

The athlete who has mono needs special attention, because there are strict guidelines for return to play in these individuals. To avoid splenic rupture, all athletes should not participate in sport activities while acutely ill from mono. Sports medicine physicians should recall that spontaneous or traumatic splenic rupture in the setting of mono usually occurs within the fourth to 21st day after the onset of clinical symptoms [45,52]. An athlete may return to easy and graduated training at 3 weeks if (1) the spleen is not palpably enlarged or painful, (2) the athlete is afebrile, (3) pharyngitis and any complications have resolved, and (4) liver enzymes are not grossly abnormal [53]. The athlete may return to contact sports and vigorous training (reconditioning necessary) at 4 weeks if these four conditions are met [53].

SUMMARY

URTIs are common acute illnesses, particularly in athletes because of the increased risk of transmission in this population. URTI management should take into account the type of illness, the potential complications of the illness, and the demand placed on the athlete to participate in practice and competition. The sports medicine physician should be armed with the latest evidence to accurately diagnose and properly treat acute URTI illness in the athlete. The overtreatment of URTIs with antibiotics, especially when not indicated, can lead to antibiotic resistance. Return-to-play decisions should be made on a case-by-case basis for the athlete and take into account the overall safety of the athlete and other teammates, coaches, and staff exposed to the athlete. The sports medicine physician represents the first line of defense in preventing, diagnosing, and managing acute URTIs in athletes and ensures the safe return of the athlete to competition.

References

[1] Woodwell DA, Cherry DK. National Ambulatory Medical Care Survey: 2002 summary, no. 346. Hyattsville (MD): National Center for Health Statistics; 2004. Advance data from vital and health statistics.

[2] Nieman DC. Current perspective on exercise immunology. Curr Sports Med Rep 2003; 2(5):239–42.

[3] Turner RB. Epidemiology, pathogenesis, and treatment of the common cold. Ann Allergy Asthma Immunol 1997;531–9.

[4] D'Alessio DJ, Peterson JA, Dick CR, et al. Transmission of experimental rhinovirus colds in volunteer married couples. J Infect Dis 1976;133:28.

[5] Kendall EJ, Bynoe ML, Tyrell DA. Virus isolations from common colds occurring in a residential school. Br Med J 1962;5297:82.

[6] Gwaltney JM Jr, Hendley JO. Transmission of experimental rhinovirus infection by contaminated surfaces. Am J Epidemiol 1982;116:828.

[7] Puhakka T, Makela M, Alanen A, et al. Sinusitis in the common cold. J Allergy Clin Immunol 1998;102:403.

[8] Teichtahl H, Buckmaster N, Pertnikovs E. The incidence of respiratory tract infection in adults requiring hospitalization for asthma. Chest 1997;112:591.

[9] Eichner ER. Infection, immunity and exercise. Phys Sports Med 1993;21(1):125–35.

[10] Arroll B, Kenealy T. Antibiotics for the common cold and acute purulent rhinitis. In: The Cochrane Library, issue 2. Chichester (UK): John Wiley & Sons, Ltd; 2005. Search date 2001.

[11] D'Agostino RB Sr, Weintraub M, Russell HK, et al. The effectiveness of antihistamines in reducing the severity of runny nose and sneezing: a meta-analysis. Clin Pharmacol Ther 1998;64:579–96.

[12] Douglas RM, Chalker EB, Treacy B. Vitamin C for preventing and treating the common cold. In: The Cochrane Library, issue 2. Chichester (UK): John Wiley & Sons, Ltd; 2005. Search date 2004.

[13] Marshall I. Zinc for the common cold. In: The Cochrane Library, issue 2. Chichester (UK): John Wiley & Sons, Ltd; 2005. Search date 1997.

[14] Caruso TJ, Gwaltney JM. Treatment of the common cold with Echinacea: a structured review. Clin Infect Dis 2005;40:807–10. Search date 2003.

[15] Kirkpatrick GL. The common cold. Prim Care 1996;23:657.

[16] Nieman DC. Physical activity, training and the immune response. Medicine & Science in Sports and Exercise 1997;29:1547–8.

[17] CDC. Centers for disease control and prevention. Nonspecific upper respiratory tract infection; 2006. Available at: cdc.gov/getsmart.

[18] Gwaltney JM Jr. Acute community-acquired sinusitis. Clin Infect Dis 1996;23:1209.

[19] Piccirillo JF. Clinical practice. Acute bacterial sinusitis. N Engl J Med 2004;351:902.

[20] Williams JW Jr, Simel DL, Roberts L, et al. Clinical evaluation for sinusitis: making the diagnosis by history and physical examination. Ann Intern Med 1992;117:705–10.

[21] Lindbaek M, Hjortdahl P. The clinical diagnosis of acute purulent sinusitis in general practice—a review. Br J Gen Pract 2002;52:491–5.

[22] Spector SL, Lotan A, English G, et al. Comparison between transillumination and x-ray in diagnosing paranasal sinus disease. J Allergy Clin Immunol 1981;67:22–6.

[23] Burke TF, Guertler AT, Timmons JH. Comparison of sinus x-rays with computed tomography scans in acute sinusitis. Acad Emerg Med 1994;1:235.

[24] Gwaltney JM Jr, Phillips CD, Miller RD, et al. Computed tomographic study of the common cold. N Engl J Med 1994;330:25.

[25] Anon JB, Jacobs MR, Poole MD, et al, for the Sinus and Allergy Health Partnership. Antimicrobial treatment guidelines for acute bacterial rhinosinusitis. [Published correction appears in Otolaryngol Head Neck Surg 2004;130:794–6]. Otolaryngol Head Neck Surg 2004;130(1 Suppl):1–45.

[26] American Academy of Pediatrics, Subcommittee on the Management of Sinusitis and Committee on Quality Improvement. Clinical practice guideline: management of sinusitis. Pediatrics 2001;108:798–808.

[27] Chow AW. Acute sinusitis: current status of etiologies, diagnosis, and treatment. Curr Clin Top Infect Dis 2001;21:31–63.

[28] Taverner D, Bickford L, Draper M. The Cochrane Collaboration. Nasal decongestants for the common cold. Cochrane database of systematic reviews. Hoboken (NJ): John Wiley and Sons; 2002.

[29] Cooper RJ, Hoffman JR, Bartlett JG, et al. Principles of appropriate antibiotic use for acute pharyngitis in adults: background. Ann Intern Med 2001;134:509.

[30] Bisno AL, Gerber MA, Gwaltney JM Jr, et al, for the Infectious Diseases Society of America. Practice guidelines for the diagnosis and management of group A streptococcal pharyngitis. Clin Infect Dis 2002;35:113–25.

[31] Centor RM, Witherspoon JM, Dalton HP, et al. The diagnosis of strep throat in adults in the emergency room. Med Decis Making 1981;1:239.

[32] NIAID. National Institute of Allergy and Infectious Diseases. Health matters: the common cold; 2004. Available at: http://www3.niaid.nih.gov/healthscience/heathtopics/colds/default.htm.

[33] Brien JH, Bass JW. Streptococcal pharyngitis: optimal site for throat culture. J Pediatr 1985;106:781.

[34] Singh M. Heated, humidified air for the common cold. In: The Cochrane Library, issue 2. Chichester (UK): John Wiley & Sons, Ltd; 2005. Search date 2003.

[35] Varonen H, Kunnamo I, Savolainen S, et al. Treatment of acute rhinosinusitis diagnosed by clinical criteria or ultrasound in primary care: a placebo-controlled randomized trial. Scand J Prim Health Care 2003;21:121–6.

[36] Kaplan EL, Top FH Jr, Dudding BA, et al. Diagnosis of streptococcal pahryngitis: differentiation of active infection from the carrier state in the symptomatic child. J Infect Dis 1971;123:490.

[37] Thomas M, Del Mar C, Glaziou P. How effective are treatments other than antibiotics for acute sore throat? Br J Gen Pract 2000;50:817–20. Search date 1999; primary sources Medline and Cochrane Controlled Trials Registry.

[38] Olympia RP, Khine H, Avner JR. Effectiveness of oral dexamethasone in the treatment of moderate to severe pharyngitis in children. Arch Pediatr Adolesc Med 2005;159:278–82.

[39] De Sutter AI, De Meyere MJ, Christiaens TC, et al. Does amoxicillin improve outcomes in patients with purulent rhinorrhea? A pragmatic randomized double-blind controlled trial in family practice. J Fam Pract 2002;51:317–23.

[40] Krober MS, Bass JW, Michels GN. Stretococcal pharyngitis: placebo-controlled double-blinded evaluation of clinical response to penicillin therapy. JAMA 1985;253:1271–4.

[41] Kelley R, Langley G, Bates L. Erythromycin: still good choice for strep throat. Clin Pediatr 1993;57:744–5.

[42] Casey JR, Pichichero M. Meta-analysis of cephalosporins versus penicillin for treatment of group A streptococcal tonsillopharyngitis in children. Pediatrics 2004a;38:866–82.

[43] Peter G. Streptococcal pharyngitis: current therapy and criteria for evaluation of new agents. Clin Infect Dis 1992;14(Suppl 2):S218–23.

[44] Snellman LW, Stang HJ, Stang JM, et al. Duration of positive throat cultures for group A streptococci after initiation of antibiotic therapy. Pediatrics 1993;911:1166–70.

[45] Rea TD, Russo JE, Katon W, et al. Prospective study of the natural history of infectious mononucleosis caused by Epstein-Barr virus. J Am Board Fam Pract 2001;14:234.

[46] Evans A, Niederman J. Epstein-Barr virus. In: Evans A, editor. Viral infections of human epidemiology and control. New York: Plenum Publishing; 1989. p. 265.

[47] Aldrete JS. Spontaneous rupture of the spleen in patients with infectious mononucleosis. Mayo Clin Proc 1992;67:910.

[48] Hosey RG, Mattacola CG, Kriss V, et al. Ultrasound assessment of spleen size in collegiate athletes. Br J Sports Med 2006;40(3):251–4.

[49] Finch SC. Laboratory findings in infectious mononucleosis. In: Carter RL, Penman HG, editors. Infectious mononucleosis. Boston: Blackwell Scientific Publications; 1969. p. 47–52.

[50] Evans AS, Niederman JC, Cenabre LC, et al. A prospective evaluation of heterophile and Epstein-Barr virus-specific IgM antibody tests in clinical and subclinical infectious mononucleosis: specificity and sensitivity of the tests and persistence of antibody. J Infect Dis 1975;132:546.

[51] Tynell E, Aurelius E, Brandell A, et al. Ayclovir and prednisolone treatment of acute infectious mononucleosis: a multicenter, double-blind, placebo-controlled study. J Infect 1996; 174:324.

[52] Torre D, Tambini R. Acyclovir for treatment of infectious mononucleosis: a meta-analysis. Scand J Infect Dis 1999;31:543.

[53] Johnson MA, Cooperberg PL, Boisvert J, et al. Spontaneous splenic rupture in infectious mononucleosis: sonographic diagnosis and follow-up. AJR Am J Roentgenol 1981; 136:111.

Clin Sports Med 26 (2007) 361–382

CLINICS IN SPORTS MEDICINE

ELSEVIER
SAUNDERS

Pulmonary and Cardiac Infections in Athletes

Roger J. Kruse, MD, FACSM[a,b], Cathy L. Cantor, MD, MBA[a,b],*

[a]Sports Care/Sports Medicine Fellowship, The Toledo Hospital, Promedica Health System, 2865 N. Reynolds Road, Suite 130, Toledo, OH 43615, USA
[b]University of Toledo, 2801 W. Bancroft, Toledo, OH 43606, USA

PNEUMONIA

Pneumonia is defined as an acute infection or inflammation of the pulmonary parenchyma. The term *community-acquired pneumonia* (CAP) is used when the patient has not been hospitalized or in a long-term facility for at least 14 days before the onset of symptoms [1]. It is estimated that 5 million cases of CAP, classified as typical or atypical, occur annually [2,3]. Typical pneumonias are most commonly caused by *Streptococcus pneumoniae* and found in very young or older patients. Atypical pneumonias are usually caused by *Legionella*, *Chlamydia*, or influenza and found most often in young adults and account for 20% to 40% of cases of CAP [4,5]. CAP is generally a serious illness with considerable morbidity and mortality, requiring increased recovery time for the athlete.

Clinical Presentation

Cough is the most common symptom in CAP. Symptoms may also include sputum production, shortness of breath, or chest pain [6,7]. Patients may present with nonspecific symptoms such as malaise, anorexia, headache, myalgias, fever, and chills [8]. Legionellosis may present with gastrointestinal symptoms such as nausea, vomiting, or diarrhea [9–11].

It is imperative to document vital signs (temperature, pulse, respiratory rate, blood pressure, and oxygen saturation) of any athlete who presents with a respiratory complaint. The vital signs on physical examination may reveal fever, tachycardia, tachypnea, hypoxemia, or hypotension [1]. The most common sign associated with CAP is fever [12]. Vital signs are important elements in the decision-making process for the appropriate management of CAP [13].

Examination may demonstrate dullness to percussion of the chest in a certain lobar distribution. Auscultation may reveal crackles, rales, or bronchial breath sounds. The patient may also exhibit increased tactile fremitus and egophony

*Corresponding author. Sports Care/Sports Medicine, 2865 N. Reynolds Road, Suite 130, Toledo, OH 43615. E-mail address: cathy.cantorMD@promedica.org (C.L. Cantor).

0278-5919/07/$ – see front matter
doi:10.1016/j.csm.2007.04.002

[1,12]. It is also important to document the patient's appearance and neurologic status [11].

Diagnosis

An infiltrate on chest radiograph is considered the "gold standard" for the diagnosis of pneumonia in the appropriate clinical scenario [8,14,15]. Other laboratory tests to consider, depending on the clinical severity, include leukocyte count, blood cultures, sputum culture with Gram stain, and urine antigens for *Streptococcus pneumoniae* and *Legionella*. The most common blood test abnormality found in CAP is leukocytosis with a leftward shift. These laboratory tests may not be indicated if the athlete is treated as an outpatient [8].

Treatment

When the diagnosis of CAP has been made, physicians must choose between inpatient or outpatient treatment for the athlete. A clinical predication tool, the pneumonia severity index, has been developed based on the likelihood of mortality of a CAP patient [13,16,17]. This index is useful for identifying patients who are at low risk of mortality from CAP and who can be safely treated as outpatients [12]. In the training room setting, the most useful indicators are vital signs and physical examination findings. The physician's clinical judgment should always override the index score.

The most common contraindications to outpatient treatment are inability to maintain oral intake, unstable vital signs, history of substance abuse, mental/cognitive impairment, or presence of comorbid conditions [12,16,18].

Because microbiologic data are not available at the time of clinical suspicion of CAP, most initial treatment regimens are empiric. Antibiotics that provide coverage against the most common organisms known to cause CAP (*Streptococcus pneumoniae*, *Mycoplasma pneumoniae*, *Chlamydia pneumoniae*, *Legionella*) should be selected. Macrolides are recommended if there are no significant risk factors for macrolide-resistant *Streptococcus pneumoniae* [18].

The American Thoracic Society (ATS) recommends not changing initial antibiotic treatment in the first 72 hours unless there is a worsening clinical situation [19]. Generally, most cases of CAP should be treated for 7 to 10 days. If atypical causes are suspected, therapy should last 10 to 14 days. The severity of the clinical presentation and the presence of coexisting illnesses should be considered in the determination of antibiotic duration [19,20].

Complications

Most patients recover from CAP without complications. One of the most common complications for the athlete is reactive airway disease. Pulmonary function tests may show decreased forced expiratory volume in 1 second (FEV_1). Transient airflow obstruction and hyper-responsiveness may be seen in these patients [21]. Up to 40% of patients may demonstrate decreased FEV_1 [22,23]. This abnormality typically resolves after 3 weeks but may last up to 2 months [22–24]. This potential complication could inhibit an athlete's full return to play. If clinically indicated, the athlete may respond to short-term inhaled bronchodilator therapy [25,26].

When the athlete has continued fever, other complications should be considered, such as pleural effusions, empyema, lung abscess, and secondary lung infection [1]. CAP patients are also susceptible to sepsis and meningitis [1].

Return to Play

Few studies are available on the amount of proper recovery time needed for athletes diagnosed with CAP. Athletes treated with an effective drug regimen usually show improvement of symptoms within 72 hours. A study by Metlay and colleagues [27] looked at time resolution of symptoms in patients who had CAP. Median time to resolution was 3 days for fever, 6 days for dyspnea, 14 days for cough, and 14 days for fatigue [27]. The athlete should be afebrile before return to training and competition. The athlete also should be re-evaluated by the team physician before clearance to assure normalcy of vital signs and respiratory status. It is recommended that exercise and training be resumed slowly when the athlete is able. For example, the first day should involve a 5- to 10-minute light elliptic or stationary bike workout. The athlete should be assessed the next day, and training may be advanced. Athletes can usually return to play sooner if they exercise early in the recovery and benefit psychologically if they see progress is being made.

ACUTE BRONCHITIS

Bronchitis is defined as inflammation of the bronchial mucous membranes. Acute bronchitis is a clinical syndrome characterized by cough (with or without sputum production) lasting up to 3 weeks, with evidence of concurrent upper airway infection [28,29]. Acute bronchitis is one of the most common conditions encountered in the primary care setting and a common ailment in the training room [29]. Acute bronchitis accounts for more than 10 million office visits yearly [30–32].

Causes

Respiratory viral infections are the most common causes of acute bronchitis. Less than 10% of patients have a bacterial etiology. The most common viruses associated with acute bronchitis include influenza A and B viruses, adenovirus, rhinovirus, parainfluenza virus, coronavirus, and respiratory synctial virus. The known bacteria that are significant agents in acute bronchitis are *Bordetella pertussis*, *Mycoplasma pneumoniae*, and *Chlamydia pneumoniae* strain TWAR [33,34]. As in CAP, the organism responsible for acute bronchitis is unlikely to be identified in the ambulatory setting. When contemplating treatment options, it is important for the physician to understand the limited role of bacterial agents in acute bronchitis. Acute bronchitis is one of the most common examples of misuse of antibiotics by the primary care physician [35].

Clinical Evaluation

Cough is the most common symptom in acute bronchitis. The patient may or may not have sputum production. Fever is unusual in acute bronchitis. If fever is present, the clinician should consider influenza or pneumonia [36,37]. The patient may also complain of concurrent or prodromal symptoms of an upper respiratory infection (URI), including pharyngitis, coryza, and fatigue [38]. Most URI symptoms improve within 5 to 7 days [39]. In acute bronchitis, the cough can last up to 3 weeks [21].

It is imperative to document vital signs (temperature, pulse, respiratory rate, blood pressure, and oxygen saturation) of any athlete who presents with a respiratory complaint. Examination often reveals findings similar to URI symtoms: pharyngeal erythema, anterior cervical lymphadenopathy, and rhinorrhea [14].

Diagnosis

The diagnosis of acute bronchitis is considered a clinical diagnosis and should be suspected in cases of acute respiratory disease with prolonged cough that continues after other signs and symptoms of acute infection have resolved [38]. It may not be necessary to obtain any further studies in the appropriate clinical situation. Abnormal vital signs (pulse >100, respiratory rate >24, or temperature >38°C) are an indication to consider further testing such as a chest radiograph. Physical examination findings on chest examination of rales on auscultation or dullness to percussion are not consistent with acute bronchitis and require further investigation [14]. Other diagnoses to consider in an athlete complaining of cough are postnasal drip, sinusitis, asthma, and gastroesophageal reflux.

Treatment

When the clinical diagnosis of acute bronchitis has been established, the recommended therapy is symptomatic. The physician may choose to use acetaminophen, ibuprofen, and nasal decongestants if appropriate. Routine antibiotic treatment of uncomplicated acute bronchitis is not recommended because the primary causes are most often viral infections [40,41]. The exception to this is in the setting of *Bordetella pertussis* infection, which is discussed in detail later.

Complications

Pulmonary function test abnormalities may also be seen in athletes who have acute bronchitis. Transient airflow obstruction and hyper-responsiveness may be seen in these patients [21]. Up to 40% of patients may demonstrate decreased FEV_1 [22,23]. This abnormality typically resolves after 3 weeks but may last up to 2 months [22–24]. This potential complication could inhibit an athlete's full return to play. If clinically indicated, the athlete may respond to short-term inhaled bronchodilator therapy [25,26]. It has been the authors' experience that athletes return to sport sooner when the reactive airway disease is treated. Athletes who have asthma or other lung conditions may have worsening symptoms.

Return to Play

There are little data regarding appropriate return-to-play guidelines for athletes who have acute bronchitis. It is important that there is proper follow-up with the team physician to ensure resolution of symptoms and to guarantee a clinical situation that does not worsen. All respiratory symptoms should be closely monitored by the athletic training staff. If the athlete's symptoms do not resolve with symptomatic treatment, then the physician should consider other diagnoses, and further workup is necessary [42].

PERTUSSIS

Bordetella pertussis, a gram-negative coccobacillus, is a commonly undiagnosed cause of acute bronchitis [43]. Pertussis, also known as whooping cough, is an acute, highly contagious infection of the respiratory airways. Pertussis is transmitted person to person by contact with aerosolized droplets [44]. One active case can infect 70% to 100% of household contacts and 50% to 80% of school contacts [45]. Because vaccine and natural immunity wane with age, pertussis has become a disease of adolescents and adults [46]. Due to the amount of time that athletes spend training together and the high infectivity of pertussis, this diagnosis must not be missed in the training room.

Clinical Presentation

The classic clinical course of pertussis is divided into three stages: catarrhal, paroxysmal, and convalescent (Box 1) [44,47,48]. Adolescents and adults may not display the typical phases of childhood infections. In adults, the disease may be characterized by a persistent cough with URI symptoms [49]. This presentation is likely to be the one encountered in the training room. Athletes may report a cough with a paroxysmal quality lasting more than 2 weeks, post-tussive emesis, or inspiratory whooping [50].

Box 1: Stages of pertussis

Catarrhal phase

Lasts 1 to 2 weeks

Most contagious phase

Clinically resembles URI

Cough increases in severity and frequency

Paroxysmal phase

Lasts 3 to 6 weeks

Clinically—spells of coughing with characteristic inspiratory whooping

Post-tussive vomiting, cyanosis, and apnea

Convalescent phase

May last 2 to 12 weeks

Cough still present

Paroxysms may recur with respiratory infection

Diagnosis

The most reliable diagnostic test for pertussis is by detection of the organism from nasopharynx secretions. The sensitivity of this test, however, is estimated to be 25% to 50% [51]. The most sensitive test (80%–100%) is polymerase chain reaction (PCR). Although PCR is a rapid and highly specific test, there is not yet a universally accepted technique. Nasopharyngeal culture is therefore recommended to make the definitive diagnosis [52]. For best yield, the nasopharyngeal swab should be inserted into the base of the nostril and remain in the posterior pharynx for 10 seconds before being withdrawn [48]. In the United States, physicians are legally required to report pertussis cases to state health department officials [53,54]. The Centers for Disease Control and Prevention (CDC) recommends that physicians report and treat pertussis when there is clinical suspicion and not wait for laboratory confirmation [54].

Treatment

In the case of proven or presumed infection, therapy should be started as soon as pertussis is suspected [28]. The recommended treatment is 2 g/d of erythromycin in four divided doses for 14 days [55,56]. If the athlete is unable to tolerate erythromycin, then two alternative regimens have shown equal efficacy: azithromycin and clarithromycin [57,58]. Azithromycin dose for adults is 500 mg in a single dose on day 1 then 250 mg per day on days 2 through 5 [59]. Clarithromycin dose for adults is 1 g per day in two divided doses for 7 days [59]. Trimethoprim-sulfamethoxazole is an additional option for those who cannot tolerate macrolides. Athletes who have confirmed or probable pertussis should be isolated for 5 days from the start of treatment [28].

Prevention

Because the vaccine and natural immunity wane with age, it is recommended to extend immunization with the tetanus toxoid–reduced diphtheria toxoid–acellular pertussis (Tdap) vaccine to the adolescent population. The CDC recommends a single dose of the Tdap vaccine (0.5 mL intramuscularly) for 11- to 18-year-olds who require a booster dose, provided they have completed the recommended primary diphtheria-tetanus-pertussis vaccine series [60,61]. The Advisory Committee of Immunization Practice also recommends a single dose of the Tdap vaccine for adults 19 to 64 years of age [59,61].

Prophylaxis

Athletes known to be in close contact with a known or suspected case of pertussis should be given prophylactic antibiotic treatment. The recommended regimen is full dosing of erythromycin for 14 days [61–63]. If erythromycin cannot be tolerated, then a 5-day course of azithromycin is acceptable [61].

Complications

Pertussis infections in the training room can lead to rapidly spreading illness among other athletes and staff. Pertussis can also cause reactive airway disease and bronchitis. Pertussis can be complicated by pneumonia, dehydration, weight loss, and sleep disturbance—all which can affect an athlete's return-to-play status and overall performance [33].

Return to Play
Athletes who have confirmed or probable pertussis should be isolated for 5 days from the start of treatment to prevent spreading the disease [28]. When reactive airway disease is involved, those symptoms should also addressed, as noted in the bronchitis section.

INFLUENZA
Influenza is an acute respiratory illness cause by influenza A or B viruses. Influenza is a common seasonal cause of acute bronchitis [41].

Clinical Presentation
The diagnosis of influenza should be considered if the athlete presents during the winter months with the abrupt onset of fever, headache, myalgias, malaise, nausea, and vomiting. These symptoms are generally accompanied by cough and sore throat [64–67].

In uncomplicated influenza, there are few physical examination findings. The health care provider in the training room should document vital signs. The patient may appear flushed. The findings may also include mild cervical lymphadenopathy and hyperemic oropharynx. The eyes may be watery or reddened [68]. Otherwise, the examination may be unremarkable. It is important to assess the athlete's hydration status and neurologic status on examination.

Diagnosis
Outpatient laboratory diagnosis of influenza can be accomplished by the detection of the virus or viral antigen in nasal washes or throat swabs [69]. The virus may also be detected from sputum samples [68]. Rapid viral diagnostic tests are available for the ambulatory setting.

Treatment
Two classes of antiviral drugs are available for the treatment of influenza [70,71]. The neuraminidase inhibitors zanamivir and oseltamivir are active against influenza A and influenza B. The M2 inhibitors amantadine and rimantidine are active against influenza A only [71]. The maximum benefit of treatment is available if given within the first 24 to 30 hours of symptoms and in patients who have fever at the time of presentation [72–74]. With appropriate treatment, the patient may have 2 to 3 days' shortening of the duration of symptoms [71].

Symptomatic treatment is also important in influenza. Acetaminophen or ibuprofen may be beneficial for fever, headache, or myalgias. The use of aspirin in pediatric patients who have influenza should be avoided due to the risk of Reye's syndrome in this population [75]. Cough suppressants may be helpful in the appropriate clinical scenario. The athlete may also benefit from inhaled bronchodilator therapy if bronchial hyper-responsiveness and decreased FEV_1 are present [33]. Athletes should be instructed to maintain proper hydration and rest during the acute illness.

Complications
Close follow-up of athletes who have severe influenza illnesses is imperative to ensure that no complications are arising. Dehydration and acute bronchitis are common complications of influenza [68]. Although rare, complications of influenza include pneumonia, myositis, rhabdomyolysis, myocarditis, encephalitis, meningitis, and Guillain-Barré syndrome [76].

Prevention
There are measures available to help prevent the illness caused by influenza. Annual vaccination is available. The currently available injectable vaccines are inactivated preparations of whole virus or split product. The whole virus vaccine is not available in the United States [72]. The United States has also made an intranasal live-attenuated vaccine available for healthy patients aged 5 to 49 years [77]. Although athletes are not on the CDC target-group list for vaccination, vaccination can be important tool to reduce the number of cases in training rooms.

Return to Play
To prevent the spread of influenza, the athlete should be kept from the training room, practices, and competitions until 5 days after the onset of symptoms. Return to full activity should be delayed until the illness has fully resolved. Athletes should be evaluated for any signs of fever, dehydration, or impaired respiratory status before full clearance.

MYOCARDITIS
Myocarditis is an inflammatory disease of the cardiac muscle that can have a wide spectrum of clinical presentations and outcomes. Myocarditis is one of the most challenging diagnoses in cardiology. Acute myocarditis can progress to dilated cardiomyopathy, heart failure, arrhythmias, and death [78]. If unrecognized in the training room, myocarditis can produce lethal results.

Causes
Myocarditis has a wide variety of infectious and noninfectious causes. The most common infectious causes are viruses. The most frequently associated viruses are coxsackievirus B, adenovirus, hepatitis C virus, cytomegalovirus, echovirus, influenza virus, and EBV. The most common causes of myocarditis found in the training room are likely viral illnesses, especially coxsackievirus B, adenovirus, and echovirus [79]. Myocarditis can also result from drug hypersensitivity, radiation, and chemical or physical agents [80,81].

Clinical Presentation
The diagnosis of myocarditis requires a high index of suspicion in the appropriate clinical setting [79]. A wide range of symptoms can be present in an athlete suffering from myocarditis. The patient may be asymptomatic or may simply give a history of a preceding URI or flu-like syndrome. The patient may also present with chest pain or symptoms of heart failure [78,79]. The athlete may present with fever, malaise, and arthralgias [82]. The diagnosis of

infective myocarditis should be considered when an athlete presents with cardiac complaints or arrhythmia issues in the course of a recognized systemic infection.

It is imperative to document vital signs in the training room. The physical examination may be normal. When the myocarditis is severe, the cardiac examination may reveal tachycardia, a muffled first heart sound along with a third heart sound, and a murmur of mitral regurgitation (MR). The examination may also reveal findings of heart failure such as edema and pulmonary crackles from fluid overload, depending on the severity of the illness. When there is associated pericarditis, a pericardial friction rub may be heard [78,79]. The examination may also reveal findings consistent with a URI.

Diagnosis

Routine blood and urine laboratory tests are generally normal in myocarditis. Cardiac enzymes may be elevated, specifically the Myoglobin binding (MB) fraction of creatine kinase (CK-MB) and troponin I [83,84]. The EKG may be normal or abnormal. The most common EKG findings are transient, nonspecific ST-T wave abnormalities. Chest radiograph findings range from normal to cardiomegaly. Pulmonary vascular congestion and edema may be exhibited in severe cases. One of the cardinal features of myocarditis can be found on echocardiography. Echocardiography may reveal decreased ventricular function. The ventricular dysfunction is generally global. Impairment of myocardial contractility may be evident on exercise-induced echocardiogram views. Echocardiography may also reveal increased left ventricular (LV) diastolic dimensions with normal septal thickness [85].

Cardiac MRI is becoming a more widely available tool to detect myocardial abnormalities. In myocarditis, the MRI may demonstrate myocardial edema and myocyte damage [86,87]. The definitive diagnosis of myocarditis is made by endomyocardial biopsy with histologic evaluation [88]. Histologic evaluation of the biopsy shows mononuclear cellular infiltrates, myocyte necrosis, and disorganized myocardiac cytoskeleton [89,90].

Treatment

Viral myocarditis is usually a self-limited disease, and treatment is generally supportive. Myocarditis, however, may progress to dilated cardiomyopathy and heart failure. Most therapy regimens are directed toward treatment of the heart failure and potential arrhythmias in serious cases [78]. Depending on the clinical situation, some patients may benefit from antiviral or immunosuppressive therapy [91–93].

Complications

Most patients who have viral myocarditis recover completely [94]; however, athletes who have viral myocarditis are at risk for heart failure, cardiomyopathy, and associated pericarditis. These athletes are also at risk for arrhythmias and sudden cardiac death [95].

Return to Play

Exercise and training can be deleterious in athletes who have myocarditis. Based on the current Bethesda Conference recommendations, athletes who have "probable or definitive evidence of myocarditis should be withdrawn from all competitive sports and undergo a prudent convalescent period of about six months following the onset of clinical manifestations" [95]. After 6 months, athletes may return to training if the following conditions are met [95]:

LV function, wall motion, and cardiac dimensions return to normal
Clinically relevant arrhythmias are absent on ambulatory Holter monitoring and graded exercise testing
Serum markers of inflammation and heart failure have normalized
The EKG has normalized

PERICARDITIS

Pericarditis (inflammation of the pericardium) may be caused by a wide variety of infectious and noninfectious processes [96,97]. Pericarditis can have a wide range of clinical presentations, from asymptomatic to severe hemodynamic compromise. Taking a careful history and knowledge of the clinical presentation of pericarditis are important in establishing the diagnosis. When the diagnosis is missed, pericarditis can become life threatening for the athlete [98].

Causes

Pericardial disease has multiple causes including infectious, neoplastic, inflammatory, degenerative, vascular, and idiopathic causes. Infectious and idiopathic causes, likely the most common causes in the training room, are found in 90% of cases of acute pericarditis [99,100]. The most common viral causes include coxsackievirus A and B, adenovirus, echovirus, and HIV. The most common bacterial causes in acute pericarditis are *Staphylococcus*, *Pneumococcus*, *Streptococcus*, *Haemophilus*, and *Neisseria* [101,102].

Clinical Presentation

The presentation of acute pericarditis varies depending on the cause. In infectious or idiopathic acute pericarditis, the major clinical symptom is chest pain. The pain in pericarditis is thought to be due to inflammation of the adjacent pleura [103]. The patient may describe the pain as retrosternal, exacerbated by coughing or deep inspiratory effort. The pain may also radiate to the back. The chest pain in acute pericarditis is often positional—worsened in the supine position and relieved by sitting upright and leaning forward [97,102,104]. The athlete may also complain of fever. Patients may also present with an associated flu-like illness with cough, fatigue, myalgias, or arthralgias [105].

It is imperative to document vital signs for athletes who have cardiac or respiratory complaints. The vitals signs may indicate severity of cardiac compromise. The pericardial friction rub is the cardinal physical sign of acute pericarditis [99]. A pericardial rub may have three components per cardiac cycle: high pitched, scratching, and grating [106]. The rub can sometimes be elicited by use of firm pressure with the stethoscope's diaphragm at the left lower sternal border of the chest wall [96,106]. The rub can often be best appreciated with the patient upright and leaning forward and is often accentuated during inspiration [107]. The physician should also look for signs of cardiac tamponade on examination: hypotension, tachycardia, jugular venous distention, and pulsus paradoxus (defined as an inspiratory systolic decrease in arterial pressure of 10 mm Hg during normal breathing) [98].

Diagnosis

Laboratory tests to consider include complete blood count, erythrocyte sedimentation rate (ESR), C-reactive protein (CRP), and cardiac enzymes. A complete blood count may illustrate increased leukocyte count [97]. Laboratory signs of inflammation including elevated ESR and CRP are commonly found in patients who have acute pericarditis. ESR and CRP are not highly specific findings because they can be elevated in multiple disease processes. Serum cardiac enzymes, CK-MB, and troponin I may also be elevated in acute pericarditis [104,108]. If the history and physical examination are appropriate, further laboratory testing should be ordered, including antinuclear antibody, tuberculin skin test, HIV serology, and blood cultures [109].

The EKG is abnormal in 90% of patients who have acute pericarditis [101,110–112]. The characteristic EKG changes found often evolve through stages. Early in pericarditis (the first few hours to days), ST-segment elevation without change in QRS morphology occurs in multiple leads. PR-segment depression may also be present. Several days later, the ST and PR segments return to baseline. This stage is followed by diffuse T-wave inversions. The EKG may normalize or the T-wave inversion may persist for weeks or months [102,104].

In acute pericarditis, the chest radiograph is generally normal; however, when at least 200 mL of pericardial effusion is present, the chest radiograph may reveal an enlarged cardiac silhouette [102]. An echocardiogram should also be obtained in patients who have suspected acute pericarditis. The echocardiogram is often normal unless there is an associated pericardial effusion [113,114].

Treatment

The physician's initial treatment decision is whether the athlete will be treated as an inpatient or an outpatient. If the athlete has simple, uncomplicated acute pericarditis and is clinically stable, then outpatient treatment with close follow-up may be appropriate [97,115]. If high-risk features are present or if the patient is clinically unstable, then inpatient treatment is recommended. High-risk features are illustrated in Box 2 [97,115].

When the clinical situation identifies a cause other than viral or idiopathic disease, specific treatment is indicated for the underlying disorder. Primary therapy goals for idiopathic or viral pericarditis are pain relief, resolution of inflammation, and resolution of effusion if present [97]. Current recommendations include the use of aspirin and other nonsteroidal anti-inflammatory drugs (NSAIDs). Colchicine may also be considered in the treatment of acute

Box 2: High-risk features in acute pericarditis

Subacute onset

Leukocytosis

Evidence of cardiac tamponade

Fever (>100.4°F)

Acute trauma

Immunosuppressed state

Large pericardial effusion without significant response to nonsteroidal anti-inflammatory drug (NSAID) treatment

History of oral anticoagulant therapy

Failure to respond to NSAID therapy within 7 days

pericarditis [116]. Corticosteroids should be considered if the patient is refractory to NSAIDs or colchicine. Close monitoring and follow-up are imperative for all athletes diagnosed with acute pericarditis.

Complications

Although pericarditis usually resolves within a few days to weeks, life-threatening complications can occur [97]. When an associated pericardial effusion is present, it may proceed to a cardiac tamponade, which is a cardiac emergency [98]. When the pericardial inflammation does not resolve, it may lead to chronic pericarditis. Chronic pericarditis may subsequently lead to constrictive pericarditis.

Return to Play

The current Bethesda Conference Guidelines recommend exclusion of the athlete who has acute pericarditis from competitive sports [95]. These athletes can return to full activity only when there is no evidence of active disease, which includes no evidence of effusion on echocardiogram and normalized serum inflammatory markers. If concurrent myocarditis is associated with acute pericarditis, then myocarditis return-to-play criteria must also be met [95].

ACUTE RHEUMATIC FEVER

Acute rheumatic fever (ARF) is an inflammatory disease that may develop after an infection with *Streptococcus* bacteria and can involve the heart, joints, skin, and brain [117]. The cardiac manifestations associated with ARF—valvulitis and carditis—can be potentially serious illnesses found in the training room. The carditis of ARF is a pancarditis that involves the pericardium, myocardium, and endocardium to varying degrees [118]. The valvulitis most frequently affects the mitral valve, aortic valve, or both [117]. Although the incidence of ARF has declined dramatically in the United States, scattered outbreaks in North America have confirmed the potentially serious consequences of this infection [119,120].

Cause

ARF results from infection with a "rheumatogenic" strain of group A streptococcus. The known serotypes associated with ARF are serotypes 1, 3, 5, 6, 14, 18, 19, 24, 27, and 29 [121]. ARF primarily affects children between age 6 and 15 years and occurs approximately 20 days after initial infection [122]. Studies have shown that an estimated 3% of individuals who have untreated group A streptococcal pharyngitis develop rheumatic fever [123].

Clinical Presentation

The clinical presentation is variable. The Jones criteria shown in Box 3 are established guidelines to aid in the diagnosis [118,124,125].

The onset of rheumatic fever follows a latent period of 7 to 35 days after a preceding group A streptococcal infection [126]. Although patients who have ARF may have any or all of the Jones criteria clinical features, the most common are polyarthritis (50%–75%) and carditis (40%–60%) [117].

On examination, the carditis is usually associated with a murmur of valvulitis [118]. The examination may reveal sinus tachycardia, an S_3 gallop, a pericardial friction rub, and cardiomegaly. The valvulitis may be characterized by a pansystolic murmur of MR, best heard at the apex, with radiation to the left axilla. The MR murmur may also be heard with or without a low-pitched mid-diastolic (Carey Coombs) murmur [127].

Diagnosis

The diagnosis of ARF is clinical but requires supporting evidence from clinical presentation and microbiologic and immunologic laboratory results. To fulfill the Jones criteria, two major criteria (or one major and two minor criteria) plus evidence of an antecedent streptococcal infection are required [118,124,125]. Throat cultures should be obtained in suspected ARF [117]. Specific antibody tests, such as antistreptolysin and anti-DNAse B should also be obtained to help confirm the diagnosis [117]. Acute phase reactants, CRP,

---

Box 3: Jones criteria

Major

Carditis

Polyarthritis

Chorea

Erythema marginatum

Subcutaneous nodules

Minor

Fever

Arthralgia

Previous rheumatic fever or rheumatic heart disease

and ESR are also usually elevated in ARF [117]. EKG and echocardiography are important diagnostic tools to assess for cardiac involvement [118,124,125]. The EKG may show prolonged PR intervals, which is a nonspecific finding [118]. The echocardiogram also reveals associated valvulitis or pericarditis, if present.

Treatment

Hospital admission is recommended for all cases to ensure complete and proper investigation. The main treatment goals are to confirm the diagnosis, treat cardiac failure, shorten the duration of symptoms, and ensure ongoing secondary prophylaxis and clinical follow-up [128]. The mainstay of treatment for ARF is NSAIDs, most commonly aspirin. Duration of NSAID treatment should be maintained until all symptoms have resolved and laboratory values are normal [129]. Depending on the severity of carditis, steroid treatment may be indicated. Antibiotic treatment with penicillin should also be given for 10 days [123]. The athlete also needs long-term antibiotic prophylaxis after the acute episode has resolved. All family contacts should be cultured and treated for streptococcal infection if indicated [123].

Complications

ARF can cause permanent cardiac damage. The mitral valve is more commonly involved than the aortic valve. Mitral stenosis (MS) is the classic finding in rheumatic heart disease and may require surgical correction [95]. Other potential complications of ARF include heart failure, myocarditis, pericarditis, arrhythmias, and endocarditis. The arrhythmia most commonly associated with MS is atrial fibrillation [117,126]. The athlete must have close monitoring and follow-up before any return to exercise.

Return to Play

If the athlete has no cardiac involvement with ARF, then after antibiotic treatment is complete and the athlete is afebrile, gradual return to play may be initiated with close physician observation (normally about 3 to 4 weeks into treatment). The athlete should also have resolution of polyarthralgias and chorea if present before return to play. Prolonged bed rest is no longer recommended after ARF [95].

All athletes who have cardiac involvement should be followed by their primary care physician, cardiologist, and dentist. When there is associated myocarditis or pericarditis, physicians should refer to the previously described return-to-play guidelines. Although MS rarely causes sudden cardiac death, careful consideration must be given if MS is present in an athlete [95]. Exercise in athletes who have MS can cause sudden increases in pulmonary capillary and pulmonary artery pressures, resulting in sudden acute pulmonary edema. It is important to assess the severity of MS at rest and during sport-related exercise with echocardiography, including measurement of pulmonary artery systolic pressure [95]. Depending on the severity of MS, the Bethesda Conference Guidelines should be followed [95].

ENDOCARDITIS

Infective endocarditis (IE) is a serious febrile infection that rapidly damages cardiac structures, spreads to extracardiac sites and, if untreated, can progress to death within weeks [130]. To avoid overlooking the diagnosis of IE, a high index of suspicion must be maintained. In the training room, the most likely case of endocarditis may be found in an athlete who has structural heart disease such as bicuspid aortic valves, mitral valve prolapse, or rheumatic heart disease.

Causes

A variety of microbial agents can cause IE. Staphylococci, streptococci, and enterococci represent most cases. The most common risk factor in athletes is structural heart disease. The skin, upper respiratory tract, and oral cavity are the primary portal of entry for streptococci and staphylococci organisms [131,132]. Bacteremia can then ensue, leading to seeding of cardiac and extracardiac sites.

Clinical Presentation

In IE, the interval between the presumed initiating bacteremia and the onset of symptoms is less than 14 days [133]. Endocarditis symptoms may develop slowly (subacute) or suddenly (acute) [134]. Fever is the most common symptom. Other common symptoms include chills, night sweats, anorexia, dyspnea, cough, chest pain, and myalgias [134]. The most common findings on physical examination are fever and a heart murmur. The murmur is usually a regurgitant heart murmur in the mitral or aortic valve position. In an athlete who has a pre-existing murmur, a new or changing murmur may be noted. Other findings on examination may include splenomegaly or cardinal peripheral manifestations such as petechiae, splinter hemorrhages, Osler's nodes, Janeway's lesions, or Roth's spots [130].

Diagnosis

The diagnosis of IE should be investigated when athletes who have fever also present with one or more of the cardinal manifestations of IE. The incorporation of clinical, laboratory, and echocardiographic data is central to the diagnosis [134,135]. Nonspecific laboratory findings may include leukocytosis and elevated ESR and CRP [135]. EKG may reveal new atrioventricular, fascicular, or bundle branch block depending on cardiac involvement [134]. The modified Duke criteria represent a diagnostic guideline for evaluating patients who have suspected IE that takes into account blood culture results, echocardiogram criteria, and history and physical examination characteristics [136].

Treatment

Treatment with parental antibiotics is usually started in the hospital but may be completed as an outpatient when the patient is afebrile and follow-up blood cultures are negative [135]. Antibiotic therapy should be selected as appropriate based on blood culture and sensitivities results. Initial therapy in native-valve IE with no history of intravenous drug abuse should be directed against streptococci organisms. Penicillin and gentamycin remain first-line therapy in this situation. Depending on the pathogen involved, antibiotic treatment should last between 2 and 6 weeks [135].

Complications

Valvular damage may lead to aortic regurgitation (AR) or MR in patients who have IE. If left untreated, IE can progress to severe heart failure and potentially fatal arrhythmias [135]. In addition, complications from septic emboli may result, such as stroke, kidney failure, or pulmonary embolism.

Return to Play

From an infectious standpoint, before return to competition, the athlete should complete at least 2 to 6 weeks of appropriate antibiotic treatment and remain afebrile with negative follow-up blood cultures. Athletes require close monitoring with frequent follow-up. When the antimicrobial treatment is complete, repeat echocardiography should be performed to establish a new baseline [135]. Repeat physical examinations are important to look for any signs of heart failure. Before any initiation of antibiotic therapy for any febrile illnesses, the athlete should have three sets of blood cultures obtained from separate sites. The athlete also requires thorough dental evaluations to ensure oral hygiene.

From a cardiac standpoint, the athlete may have residual MR or AR. Athletes who have MR from IE may be restricted from competition. Current recommendations are based on the severity of MR, echocardiogram findings of LV size and function, and pulmonary artery pressure readings [95]:

> Athletes who have mild to moderate MR in normal sinus rhythm, with normal LV size, LV function, and pulmonary artery pressures, can participate in all competitive sports.
> Athletes who have mild LV enlargement (<60 mm) may participate but are restricted to certain classes of sports.
> Athletes who have severe MR, LV enlargement (>60 mm), LV systolic dysfunction, or elevated pulmonary artery pressures should not participate in any competitive sports.

If AR is present in any athlete who has IE, the current recommendations are to assess the severity of AR with echocardiography and measurement of LV end diastolic size [95]:

> Athletes who have mild to moderate AR and normal LV end diastolic size may participate in all competitive sports.
> Athletes who have severe AR and increased LV diastolic diameter (>65 mm) should not participate in sports.
> Symptomatic athletes who have mild to moderate AR should not participate in sports regardless of LV size.

SUMMARY

Pulmonary and cardiac infections in the athlete can have a wide range of presentations and complications. These infections may present few problems for the training athlete or become life-threatening. The team physician must be able to recognize the diagnosis, give the appropriate treatment, understand the potential complications, and ensure proper follow-up and return-to-play protocols.

References

[1] Baldwin DR, Macfarlane JT. Community-acquired pneumonia. In: Cohen J, Powderly WG, editors. Cohen & Powderly: infectious diseases. 2nd edition. St. Louis (MO): Mosby; 2004. p. 369–80.

[2] File TM Jr. The epidemiology of respiratory tract infections. Semin Respir Infect 2000;15: 184–94.

[3] Bartlett JG, Breiman RF, Mandell LA. Community-acquired pneumonia in adults: guidelines for management. Clin Infect Dis 1998;26:811–38.

[4] Gleason PP, Meehan TP, Fine JM, et al. Associations between initial antimicrobial therapy and medical outcomes for hospitalized elderly patients with pneumonia. Arch Intern Med 1999;159:2562–72.

[5] Houck PM, MacLehose RF, Niederman MS, et al. Empiric antibiotic therapy and mortality among Medicare pneumonia inpatients in 10 western states: 1993, 1995, and 1997. Chest 2001;119:1420–6.

[6] Fine MJ, Smith MA, Carson CA, et al. Prognosis and outcomes of patients with community-acquired pneumonia. A meta-analysis. JAMA 1996;275:134–41.

[7] Woodhead MA, Macfarlane JT. Comparative clinical and laboratory features of legionella with pneumococcal and mycoplasma pneumonia. Br J Dis Chest 1987;81:133–9.

[8] Bartlett JG, Mundy LM. Community acquired pneumonia. N Engl J Med 1995;333: 1618–24.

[9] Fraser DW, Tsai T, Ornstein W, et al. Legionnaires' disease: description of an epidemic of pneumonia. N Engl J Med 1977;297:1189–97.

[10] Mulazimoglu L, Yu VL. Can Legionnaires disease be diagnosed by clinical criteria? A critical review. Chest 2001;120:1049–53.

[11] Yu VL, Kroboth FJ, Shonnard J, et al. Legionnaires' disease: new clinical perspective from a prospective pneumonia study. Am J Med 1982;73:357–61.

[12] Marrie TJ. Community-acquired pneumonia. Clin Infect Dis 1994;18:501–15.

[13] Fine MJ, Hough LJ, Medsger AR, et al. The hospital admission decision for patients with community-acquired pneumonia. Arch Intern Med 1997;157:36–44.

[14] Metlay JP, Kapoor WN, Fine MJ. Does this patient have community-acquired pneumonia? Diagnosing pneumonia by history and physical examination. JAMA 1997;278:1440–5.

[15] Mandell LA, Bartlett JG, Dowell SF, et al. Update of practice guidelines for the management of community-acquired pneumonia in immunocompetent adults. Clin Infect Dis 2003;37: 1405–33.

[16] Farr BM, Sloman AJ, Fisch MJ. Predicting death in patients hospitalized for community-acquired pneumonia. Ann Intern Med 1991;115:428–36.

[17] Fine MJ, Singer DE, Hanusa BH, et al. Validation of a pneumonia prognostic index using the MedisGroups Comparative Hospital Database. Am J Med 1993;94:153–9.

[18] Niederman MS, Bass JB Jr, Campbell GD, et al. Guidelines for the initial management of adults with community-acquired pneumonia: diagnosis, assessment of severity, and initial antimicrobial therapy. Am Rev Respir Dis 1993;148:1418–26.

[19] Niederman MS, Mandell LA, Anzueto A, et al. Guidelines for the management of adults with community-acquired pneumonia. Diagnosis, assessment of severity, antimicrobial therapy, and prevention. Am J Respir Crit Care Med 2001;163:1730–54.

[20] File TM. Community-acquired pneumonia. Lancet 2003;362:1991–2001.

[21] Boldy DA, Skidmore SJ, Ayres JG. Acute bronchitis in the community: clinical features, infective factors, changes in pulmonary function and bronchial reactivity to histamine. Respir Med 1990;84:377–85.

[22] Williamson HA Jr. Pulmonary function tests in acute bronchitis: evidence for reversible airway obstruction. J Fam Pract 1987;25:251–6.

[23] Melbye H, Kongerud J, Vorland L. Reversible airflow limitation in adults with respiratory infection. Eur Respir J 1994;7:1239–45.

[24] Hueston WJ. A comparison of albuterol and erythromycin for the treatment of acute bronchitis. J Fam Pract 1991;33:476–80.

[25] Hueston WJ. Albuterol delivered by metered-dose inhaler to treat acute bronchitis. J Fam Pract 1994;39:437–40.

[26] Melbye H, Aasebo U, Straume B. Symptomatic effect of inhaled fenoterol in acute bronchitis: a placebo-controlled double-blind study. Family Practice 1991;8:216–22.

[27] Metlay JP, Schulz R, Li Y, et al. Influence of age on symptoms and presentation in patients with community acquired pneumonia. Arch Intern Med 1997;157(13):1453–4.

[28] Braman SS. Chronic cough due to chronic bronchitis: ACCP evidence-based clinical practice guidelines. Chest 2006;129:104S–15S.

[29] Anish EJ. Lower respiratory tract infections in adults. Clinics in Family Practice 2004;6(1): 75–99.

[30] Mannino D, Homa D, Akinbami L, et al. Chronic obstructive pulmonary disease surveillance: United States, 1971–2000. MMWR Morb Mortal Wkly Rep 2002;51:1–13.

[31] Mannino D, Gagnon R, Petty T, et al. Obstructive lung disease and low lung function in adults in the United States: data from the National Health and Nutrition Examination Survey, 1988–1994. Arch Intern Med 2000;160:1683–9.

[32] Irwin RS, Rosen MJ, Braman SS. Cough: a comprehensive review. Arch Intern Med 1977;137:1186–91.

[33] Gonzales R, Sande MA. Uncomplicated acute bronchitis. Ann Intern Med 2000;133: 981–91.

[34] Gwaltney JM. Acute bronchitis. In: Mandel GL, Bennett JE, Dolin R, editors. Mandell, Douglas, and Bennet's principles and practice of infectious diseases. Philadelphia: Churchill Livingstone; 2000. p. 703–6.

[35] Gonzales R, Steiner JF, Lum A, et al. Decreasing antibiotic use in ambulatory practice: impact of a multidimensional intervention on the treatment of uncomplicated acute bronchitis in adults. JAMA 1999;281:1512–9.

[36] Irwin RS, Curley FJ, French CL. Chronic cough. The spectrum and frequency of causes, key components of the diagnostic evaluation, and outcome of specific therapy. Am Rev Respir Dis 1990;141:640–7.

[37] Mello CJ, Irwin RS, Curley FJ. Predictive values of character, timing and complications of chronic cough in diagnosing its cause. Arch Intern Med 1996;156:997–1003.

[38] Evans AS. Clinical syndromes in adults caused by respiratory infection. Med Clin North Am 1967;51:803–18.

[39] Heikkinen T, Jarvinen A. The common cold. Lancet 2003;361:51–9.

[40] Snow V, Mottur-Pilson C, Gonzales R. Principles of appropriate antibiotic use for treatment of acute bronchitis in adults. Ann Intern Med 2001;134:518–20.

[41] Gonzales R, Bartlett JG, Besser RE, et al. Principles of appropriate antibiotic use for treatment of uncomplicated acute bronchitis: background. Ann Intern Med 2001;134: 521–9.

[42] Irwin RS, Boulet LP, Cloutier MM. Managing cough as a defense mechanism and as a symptom. A consensus panel report of the American College of Chest Physicians. Chest 1998; 114:133S–81S.

[43] Cherry JD. Epidemiological, clinical, and laboratory aspects of pertussis in adults. Clin Infect Dis 1999;28(Suppl 2):S112–7.

[44] Tozzi AE, Celentano LP, Atti ML, et al. Diagnosis and management of pertussis. Can Med Assoc J 2005;172(4):509–15.

[45] Atkinson W. Epidemiology and prevention of vaccine preventable diseases. Atlanta (GA): Centers for Disease Control and Prevention; 1996.

[46] Bass JW, Klenk EL, Kotheimer JB, et al. Antimicrobial treatment of pertussis. J Pediatr 1969;75:768–81.
[47] Mattoo S, Cherry JD. Molecular pathogenesis, epidemiology, and clinical manifestations of respiratory infections due to Bordetella pertussis and other Bordetella subspecies. Clin Microbiol Rev 2005;18:326–82.
[48] Centers for Disease Control and Prevention. Guidelines for the control of pertussis outbreaks. 2000 (amendments made in 2005 and 2006). Available at: http://www.cdc.gov/nip/publications/pertussis/guide.htm. Accessed November 1, 2006.
[49] Wright SW, Edwards KM, Decker MD, et al. Pertussis infection in adults with persistent cough. JAMA 1995;273:1044–6.
[50] Brown MO, St. Anna L, Ohl M. Clinical inquiries. What are the indications for evaluating a patient with cough for pertussis? J Fam Pract 2005;54:74–6.
[51] Anonymous. Case definitions. Pertussis (whooping cough). Epidemiol Bull 1999;20:13–4.
[52] Muller FM, Hoppe JE, Wirsing von Konig CH. Laboratory diagnosis of pertussis: state of the art in 1997. J Clin Microbiol 1997;35:2435–43.
[53] Hopkins RS, Jajosky RA, Hall PA, et al. Centers for Disease Control and Prevention. Summary of notifiable diseases—United States, 2003. MMWR Morb Mortal Wkly Rep 2005;52:1–85.
[54] Roush S, Birkhead G, Koo D, et al. Mandatory reporting of diseases and conditions by health care professionals and laboratories. JAMA 1999;282:164–70.
[55] Bergquist SO, Bernander S, Dahnsjo H. Erythromycin in the treatment of pertussis: a study of bacteriologic and clinical effects. Pediatr Infect Dis J 1987;6:458–61.
[56] Centers for Disease Control and Prevention. Prevention and control of influenza: recommendations of the Advisory Committee on Immunization Practices (ACIP). MMWR Recomm Rep 1999;48:1–28.
[57] Langley JM, Halperin SA, Boucher FD. Azithromycin is as effective as and better tolerated than erythromycin estolate for the treatment of pertussis. Pediatrics 2004;114:e96–101.
[58] Aoyama T, Sunakawa K, Iwata S. Efficacy of short-term treatment of pertussis with clarithromycin and azithromycin. J Pediatr 1996;129:761–4.
[59] Powell KR, Baltimore RS, Bernstein HH, et al. Prevention of pertussis among adolescents: recommendations for use of tetanus toxoid, reduced diphtheria toxoid, and acellular pertussis (Tdap) vaccine. Pediatrics 2006;117:965–78.
[60] Anonymous. Adacel and Boostrix: Tdap vaccines for adolescents and adults. Med Lett Drugs Ther 2006;48:5–6.
[61] Centers for Disease Control and Prevention. Recommended antimicrobial agents for treatment and postexposure prophylaxis of pertussis: 2005 CDC guidelines. MMWR Morb Mort Wkly Rep 2005;54(RR–14):1–16.
[62] Kerr JR, Preston NW. Current pharmacotherapy of pertussis. Expert Opin Pharmacother 2001;2:1275–82.
[63] Abramowicz M. The choice of antibacterial drugs. Med Lett Drugs Ther 2001;43:69–78.
[64] Smith N, Bresee JS, Shay DK, et al. Prevention and control of influenza: recommendations of the advisory committee on immunization practices. MMWR Morb Mortal Recomm Rep 2006;55:1–42.
[65] Hayden FG, Fritz R, Lobo MC, et al. Local and systemic cytokine responses during experimental human influenza A virus infection. Relation to symptom formation and host defense. J Clin Invest 1998;101:643–9.
[66] Hall CB, Douglas RG Jr. Nosocomial influenza infection as a cause of intercurrent fevers. Pediatrics 1975;55:673–7.
[67] Pope JS, Koenig SM. Pulmonary disorders in the training room. Clin Sports Med 2005;24:541–64.

[68] Treanor JJ. Influenza virus. In: Mandell GL, Bennett JE, Dolin R, editors. Principles and practice of infectious disease. 6th edition. Philadelphia: Churchill Livingstone; 2005. p. 2060–78.

[69] Call SA, Vollenweider MA, Hornung CA, et al. Does this patient have influenza? JAMA 2005;293:987–97.

[70] Stiver G. The treatment of influenza with antiviral drugs. CMAJ 2003;168:49–56.

[71] Abramowicz M. Antiviral drugs for prophylaxis and treatment of influenza. Med Lett Drugs Ther 2005;47:93–5.

[72] Hayden FG, Osterhaus AD, Treanor JJ, et al. Efficacy and safety of the neuraminidase inhibitor zanamivir in the treatment of influenzavirus infections. N Engl J Med 1997;337: 874–80.

[73] Campion K, Silagy C, Cooper C, et al. Randomised trial of efficacy and safety of inhaled zanamivir in treatment of influenza A and B virus infections. The MIST (Management of Influenza in the Southern Hemisphere Trialists) Study Group. Lancet 1998;352: 1877–91.

[74] Nicholson KG, Aoki FY, Osterhaus ADME, et al. Efficacy and safety of oseltamivir in treatment of acute influenza: a randomized controlled trial. Lancet 2000;355:1845–50.

[75] Waldman RJ, Hall WN, McGee H, et al. Aspirin as a risk factor in Reye's syndrome. JAMA 1982;247:3089–94.

[76] Hayden FG. Influenza. In: Goldman L, Ausiello D, editors. Cecil textbook of medicine. 22nd edition. St. Louis (MO): Saunders; 2004. p. 1974–87.

[77] Cooper NJ, Sutton AJ, Abrams KR, et al. Effectiveness of neuraminidase inhibitors in treatment and prevention of influenza A and B: systematic review and meta-analyses of randomized controlled trials. BMJ 2003;326:1235–42.

[78] Wynne J, Braunwald E, et al. The cardiomyopathies and myocarditides. In: Braunwald E, Fauci A, Kasper D, editors. Harrison's principles of internal medicine. 15th edition. New York: McGraw Hill; 2001. p. 1359–65.

[79] Feldman AM McNamara D. Myocarditis. N Engl J Med 2000; 343:1388–98.

[80] Bowles NE, Ni J, Kearney DL, et al. Detection of viruses in myocardial tissues by polymerase chain reaction. Evidence of adenovirus as a common cause of myocarditis in children and adults. J Am Coll Cardiol 2003;42:466–72.

[81] Kuhl U, Pauschinger M, Seeberg B, et al. Viral persistence in the myocardium is associated with progressive cardiac dysfunction. Circulation 2005;112:1965–70.

[82] See DM, Tilles JG. Viral myocarditis. Rev Infect Dis 1991;13:951–6.

[83] Karjalainen J. Clinical diagnosis of myocarditis and dilated cardiomyopathy. Scand J Infect Dis 1993;88(Suppl):33–43.

[84] Babuin L, Jaffe AS. Troponin: the biomarker of choice for the detection of cardiac injury. Can Med Assoc J 2005;173(10):1191–202.

[85] Felker GM, Boehmer JP, Hruban RH, et al. Echocardiographic findings in fulminant and acute myocarditis. J Am Coll Cardiol 2000;36:227–32.

[86] Gagliardi MG, Bevilacqua M, Renzi P, et al. Usefulness of magnetic resonance imaging for diagnosis of acute myocarditis in infants and children, and comparison with endomyocardial biopsy. Am J Cardiol 1991;68:1089–91.

[87] Marcu CB, Beek AM, Van Rossum AC. Clinical applications of cardiovascular magnetic resonance imaging. Can Med Assoc J 2006;175:911–7.

[88] O'Connell JB, Mason JW. Diagnosing and treating active myocarditis. West J Med 1989;150:431–5.

[89] Mason JE. Techniques for right and left ventricular endomyocardial biopsy. Am J Cardiol 1978;41:887–92.

[90] Abelmann WH, Baim DS, Schnitt SJ. Endomyocardial biopsy: is it of clinical value? Postgrad Med J 1992;68(Suppl 1):S44–6.

[91] Monrad ES, Matsumori A, Murphy JC, et al. Therapy with cyclosporine in experimental murine myocarditis with encephalomyocarditis virus. Circulation 1986;73:1058–64.

[92] Tomioka N, Kishimoto C, Matsumori A, et al. Effects of prednisolone on acute viral myocarditis in mice. J Am Coll Cardiol 1986;7:868–72.

[93] Magnani JW, Dec GW. Myocarditis: current trends in diagnosis and treatment. Circulation 2006;113:876–90.

[94] Remes J, Helin M, Vaino P, et al. Clinical outcome and left ventricular function 23 years after acute coxsackie virus myopericarditis. Eur Heart J 1990;11:182–8.

[95] Maron BJ, Zipes DP, Ackerman MJ, et al. 36th Bethesda Conference: eligibility recommendations for competitive athletes with cardiovascular abnormalities. J Am Coll Cardiol 2005;45:1313–75.

[96] Braunwald E, et al. Pericardial disease. In: Braunwald E, Fauci A, Kasper D, editors. Harrison's principles of internal medicine. 15th edition. New York: McGraw Hill; 2001. p. 1365–72.

[97] Lange RA, Hillis D. Acute pericarditis. N Engl J Med 2004;351:2195–201.

[98] Spodick DH. Acute cardiac tamponade. N Engl J Med 2003;349:684–90.

[99] Zayas R, Anguita M, Torres F, et al. Incidence of specific etiology and role of methods for specific etiologic diagnosis of primary acute pericarditis. Am J Cardiol 1995;75:378–82.

[100] Permanyer-Miralda G, Sagrista-Sauleda J, Soler-Soler J. Primary acute pericardial disease: a prospective series of 231 consecutive patients. Am J Cardiol 1985;56:623–30.

[101] Spodick DH. Pericardial diseases. In: Braunwald E, Zipes DP, Libby P, editors. Heart disease, a textbook of cardiovascular medicine. 6th edition. Philadelphia: WB Saunders; 2001. p. 1823–76.

[102] Troughton RW, Asher CR, Klein AL. Pericarditis. Lancet 2004;363:717–27.

[103] Lee TH, et al. Chest discomfort and palpitations. In: Braunwald E, Fauci A, Kasper D, editors. Harrison's principles of internal medicine. 15th edition. New York: McGraw Hill; 2001. p. 60–6.

[104] Spodick DH. Acute pericarditis: current concepts and practice. JAMA 2003;289:1150–3.

[105] Smith WG. Coxsackie B myopericarditis in adults. Am Heart J 1970;80:34–46.

[106] Spodick DH. Pericardial rub. Prospective, multiple observer investigation of pericardial friction in 100 patients. Am J Cardiol 1975;35:357–62.

[107] O'Rourke RA, Braunwald E, et al. Physical examination of the cardiovascular system. In: Braunwald E, Fauci A, Kasper D, editors. Harrison's principles of internal medicine. 15th edition. New York: McGraw Hill; 2001. p. 1255–62.

[108] Bonnefoy E, Godon P, Kirkorian G, et al. Serum cardiac troponin I and ST-segment elevation in patients with acute pericarditis. Eur Heart J 2000;21:832–6.

[109] Permanyer-Miralda G. Acute pericardial disease: approach to the aetiologic diagnosis. Heart 2004;90:252–4.

[110] Shabetai R. Function of the pericardium. In: Fowler NO, editor. The pericardium in health and disease. Mount Kisco (NY): Futura; 1985. p. 19–50.

[111] Shabetai R. Acute pericarditis. Cardiol Clin 1990;8:639–44.

[112] Spodick DH. Electrocardiogram in acute pericarditis. Distributions of morphologic and axial changes by stages. Am J Cardiol 1974;33:470–4.

[113] Cheitlin MD, Alpert JS, Armstrong WF, et al. ACC/AHA guidelines for the clinical application of echocardiography: a report of the American College of Cardiology/American Heart Association Task Force on Practice Guidelines (Committee on Clinical Application of Echocardiography): developed in collaboration with the American Society of Echocardiography. Circulation 1997;95:1686–744.

[114] Cheitlin MD, Armstrong WF, Aurigemma GP, et al. ACC/AHA/ASE 2003 guideline update for the clinical application of echocardiography: summary article: a report of the American College of Cardiology/American Heart Association Task Force on Practice Guidelines (ACC/AHA/ASE Committee to Update the 1997 Guidelines for the Clinical Application of Echocardiography). Circulation 2003;108:1146–62.

[115] Imazio M, Demichelis B, Parrini I, et al. Day-hospital treatment of acute pericarditis: a management program for outpatient therapy. J Am Coll Cardiol 2004;43:1042–6.

[116] Imazio M, Bobbio M, Cecchi E, et al. Colchicine as first-choice therapy for recurrent pericarditis: results of the CORE (COlchicine for REcurrent pericarditis) trial. Arch Intern Med 2005;165:1987–91.

[117] Carapetis JR. Rheumatic fever. In: Cohen J, Powderly WG, editors. Cohen & Powderly: infectious diseases. 2nd edition. St. Louis (MO): Mosby; 2004. p. 669–76.

[118] Dajanii AS, Ayoub E, Bierman FZ, et al. Guidelines for the diagnosis of rheumatic fever. Jones criteria, 1992 update. Special writing group of the Committee on Rheumatic Fever, Endocarditis, and Kawasaki Disease of the Council on Cardiovascular Disease in the Young of the American Heart Association. JAMA 1992;268:2069–73.

[119] Veasy LG, Tani LY, Hill HR. Persistence of acute rheumatic fever in the intermountain area of the United States. J Pediatr 1994;124:9–16.

[120] Johnson DR, Stevens DL, Kaplan EL. Epidemiologic analysis of group A streptococcal serotypes associated with severe systemic infections, rheumatic fever, or uncomplicated pharyngitis. J Infect Dis 1992;166:374–82.

[121] Stollerman GH. Rheumatogenic streptococci and autoimmunity. Clin Immunol Immunopathol 1991;61:131–42.

[122] Carapetis JR, Currie BJ. Rheumatic fever in a high-incidence population: the importance of monoarthritis and low-grade fever. Arch Dis Child 2001;85:223–7.

[123] Dajanii AS, Bisno AL, Chung KJ, et al. Special report on the prevention of rheumatic fever. A statement for health professionals by the Committee on Rheumatic Fever, Endocarditis, and Kawasaki Disease of the Council on Cardiovascular Disease in the Young of the American Heart Association. Circulation 1988;78:1082–6.

[124] Jones TD. The diagnosis of rheumatic fever. JAMA 1944;126:481–4.

[125] Stollerman GH, Markowitz M, Taranta A, et al. Jones criteria (revised) for guidance in the diagnosis of rheumatic fever. Circulation 1965;32:664–8.

[126] Stollerman GH. Rheumatic fever. Lancet 1997;349:935–42.

[127] Anonymous. Rheumatic fever and rheumatic heart disease—report of a WHO study group. World Health Organization Technical Report Series (764). Geneva (Switzerland): World Health Organization; 1988. p. 1–58.

[128] Albert DA, Harel L, Karrison T. The treatment of rheumatic carditis: a review and meta-analysis. Medicine 1995;74:1–12.

[129] Gibofsky A, Zabriskie J. Acute rheumatic fever and poststreptococcal arthritis. In: Harris ED, Budd RC, Genovese MC, editors. Kelley's textbook of rheumatology. 7th edition. St. Louis (MO): Saunders; 2005. p. 1689–99.

[130] Karchmer AW, et al. Infective endocarditis. In: Braunwald E, Fauci A, Kasper D, editors. Harrison's principles of internal medicine. 15th edition. New York: McGraw Hill; 2001. p. 809–20.

[131] Jalal S, Khan KA, Alai MS, et al. Clinical spectrum of infective endocarditis: 15 years experience. Indian Heart J 1998;50:516–9.

[132] Choudhury R, Grover A, Varma J, et al. Active infective endocarditis observed in an Indian hospital 1981–1991. Am J Cardiol 1992;70:1453–8.

[133] Karchmer AW. Infections of prosthetic heart valves. In: Waldvogel F, Bisno AL, editors. Infections associated with indwelling medical devices. Washington, DC: American Society for Microbiology; 2000. p. 145–72.

[134] Mylonakis E, Calderwood SB. Infective endocarditis in adults. N Engl J Med 2001;345:1318–28.

[135] Baddour LM, Wilson WR, Bayer AS, et al. AHA scientific statement on infective endocarditis—diagnosis, antimicrobial therapy, and management of complications. Circulation 2005;e394–428.

[136] Durack DT, Lukes AS, Bright KD, et al. New criteria for diagnosis of infective endocarditis: utilization of specific echocardiographic findings. Am J Med 1994;96:200–9.

Clin Sports Med 26 (2007) 383–396

CLINICS IN SPORTS M

ELSEVIER
SAUNDERS

Bacterial Dermatoses in

Peter E. Sedgwick, MD[a],*, William W.
Christina T. Smith, MD[c]

[a]Sports Medicine Program, Maine Medical Center, 272 Congress Street,
Portland, ME 04101, USA
[b]Family Practice Residency Program, Maine Medical Center,
272 Congress Street, Portland, ME 04101, USA
[c]Sports Medicine Institute, 250 Cetronia Road, Allentown, PA 18104, USA

B acterial skin dermatoses are common in athletes, and it is the role of any team physician to be able to recognize and treat such problems. Despite the skin's role as an efficient barrier, a moist environment coupled with frequent skin trauma and athlete contact with equipment and other players predispose to acquiring infections. Many of these infections are easily treated and relatively benign, but in the past 10 years, there has been a dramatic rise in methicillin-resistant *Staphylococcus aureus* (MRSA) infections. These infections can be disfiguring or even potentially life threatening if not treated promptly and appropriately. After discussion of community-acquired MRSA infections among athletes, this article focuses on the recognition of, management of, and return-to-play guidelines for common bacterial skin infections in athletes. Some of the more unusual bacterial infections that may present in this population are also reviewed.

METHICILLIN-RESISTANT *STAPHYLOCOCCUS AUREUS*
Prevalence of Community-Acquired Methicillin-Resistant *Staphylococcus aureus*

Although MRSA infections have been a complication in hospital settings for over 40 years [1], first emerging in the United States in 1968 [2], the emergence of community-acquired MRSA infections in sport has become a reality in the past several years. Traditional risk factors for MRSA infections do not apply to the community-acquired MRSA population, because these individuals tend to be immunocompetent and often do not have a history of recent antibiotic use. The actual prevalence of community-acquired MRSA varies widely with population and geography [2]. Collecting data from 2001 to 2002, an National Health and Nutrition Examination Survey study of nasal carriage in 9622 subjects found a 32.4% prevalence of methicillin-sensitive *Staphylococcus aureus* (MSSA) when culturing anterior nares versus only 0.84% prevalence of

*Corresponding author. E-mail address: sedgwp@gmail.com (P.E. Sedgwick).

0278-5919/07/$ – see front matter
doi:10.1016/j.csm.2007.04.008

olonization [3]. This statistic, however, captures only a snapshot in whereas many MRSA and MSSA colonizations are thought to be tran- and do not necessarily lead to or indicate infection. Although *Staphylococcus eus* can infect the bloodstream, bone, heart, lung, and meninges, it is the skin and soft tissue infections that are most commonly seen in the athletic setting [4]. Among sports teams, there have been multiple studies showing high rates of carriage and of infection [5–7]. Figures range from 9% carriage on a football team [5] to 27% on a wrestling team [7].

When an athlete is a carrier or is infected, teammates and opponents in contact are at risk. It has been shown that there are limited serotypes of the bacteria among teams and often within leagues, suggesting a high rate of transmission among players within a team and between teams [5,7]. Implementing stringent disinfection and quarantine, providing education, and following return-to-play guidelines described in the following sections may decrease the incidence of these transmissions [8].

Clinical Features of Community-Acquired Methicillin-Resistant
Staphylococcus aureus

Although community-acquired MRSA infections can infect any athlete, there is an increased risk of infections among teammates who are sharing equipment. Often, infections occur at turf-abrasion sites or other areas of open skin [5]. These infections have a predilection for causing soft tissue abscesses. Studies have been done on environmental surfaces, whirlpools, taping gel, and other training room equipment, with variable results, but there is still no reproducible microbial link to such equipment [5]. Better hygiene practices have improved infection rates, however. All abscesses in athletes and any skin infections that are nonresponsive to standard antibiotic therapy should be suspected for community-acquired MRSA [7].

Management of Community-Acquired Methicillin-Resistant
Staphylococcus aureus

When MRSA is suspected by history, by appearance of the lesion, or by knowledge of an infected team member, it is important to obtain a culture of the wound and to treat presumptively with appropriate antibiotics. Local wound care alone such as incision and drainage of an abscess may be sufficient in an immunocompetent host, but most recommendations also include systemic antibiotics. Trimethoprim/sulfamethoxazole DS (160TMP/800SMX) twice daily or doxycycline (100 mg) twice daily are good first-line agents, and 10 days to 2 weeks is the recommended duration for treatment. Clindamycin (300 mg) four times daily for 10 to 14 days or linezolid (600 mg) every 12 hours for 10 to 14 days are valid second-line agents but should be used with caution due to high levels of inducible resistance. In more severe or systemic illnesses, intravenous therapy with vancomycin (dose is variable depending on measured serum levels) should be used for 14 days. Antibiotic regimens for MRSA infections are summarized in Table 1. Conflicting reports exist on decontamination treatment of MRSA carriers. A Cochrane review of six

Table 1
Guidelines for treatment of superficial methicillin-resistant *Staphylococcus aureus* skin infections

Antibiotic	Dose[a]	Duration
First-line		
Trimethoprim/sulfamethoxazole	160TMP/800SMX	po bid × 10–14 d
Doxycycline	100 mg	po bid × 10–14 d
Alternative		
Clindamycin	300 mg	po qid × 10–14 d
Linezolid	600 mg	po q 12 h × 10–14 d

Susceptibility of methicillin-resistant *Staphylococcus aureus* infection may vary with region and time. Any evidence of systemic infection warrants hospitalization with intravenous vancomycin therapy.
[a]Adult doses provided.

randomized controlled trials found no difference in decolonization rates with antibiotics (nasal mupirocin, oral antibiotics, or both) in four of six trials [9]. More studies are needed for definitive recommendations about decontamination treatment.

IMPETIGO

Description and Diagnosis

Impetigo, one of the most common bacterial infections of athletes, is characterized by superficial skin infections caused by *Streptococcus* or *Staphylococcus* species, or a combination of the two. Lesions are highly contagious and notorious for spreading among children and adolescents in close settings such as teams or camps. Often, insect bites or skin breaks may be the source of infection, but unbroken skin is more commonly present. Palms and soles are rarely affected [10].

"Honey-crusted" lesions are classic (Fig. 1), but there can be a variable presentation of infection. Lesions frequently start as isolated vesicular or pustular lesions but usually progress to one of two forms: bullous and nonbullous [11]. There has been an attempt to characterize differing bacterial etiologies to the different forms of impetigo, but it is now recognized that this is not usually the case [10]. Although systemic manifestations are rare, postinfectious pyelonephritis can occur and has been reported with strains among contaminated rugby players [12]. Adenopathy may or may not be present near sites of the lesion.

Differential Diagnosis

Bullous impetigo may resemble contact dermatitis such as poison ivy, Stevens-Johnson syndrome, or thermal burns [13]. Nonbullous lesions can be difficult to assess early in the course and may mimic acne, tinea, dermatophytes, or herpes simplex virus [14].

Treatment and Return to Play

Due to the highly contagious nature of the disease, impetigo warrants a high level of intervention in treatment and prevention of spread. MRSA is also of

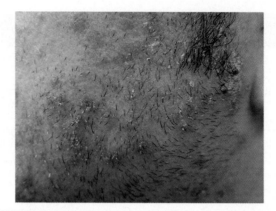

Fig. 1. Classic honey-crusted lesions of impetigo. (*Courtesy of* Daniel L. Stulberg, MD, Denver, CO.)

high concern because prevalence is increasing dramatically among athletes. Topical treatment with mupirocin (Bactroban) twice daily for 10 days is recommended for limited infections (Table 2). Systemic treatment with a first-generation cephalosporin (eg, cephalixin, 500 mg orally four times a day for 7 days) or macrolide (eg, azithromycin, 500 mg orally for 1 day, then 250 mg orally for 4 days) may be warranted as adjunctive therapy in addition to topical therapy for non-MRSA cases covering large areas of the body [15]. Topical treatment must start in all cases with removal of the lesions' crusts by soaking, because topical therapy without such removal is ineffective.

Return-to-play guidelines for all suspected staphylococcal or streptococcal skin infections (impetigo, folliculitis, furuncles, carbuncles, abscesses, erysipelas, and cellulitis) are grouped together in most guidelines (Table 3). The National Collegiate Athletic Association guidelines for wrestling are the most comprehensive and restrictive, recommending return to practice or play only if players: (1) have no new lesions within the past 48 hours, (2) have completed 72 hours of antibiotic treatment, and (3) have no moist, exudative, or draining lesions at tournament or practice [16]. The National Federation of High Schools has similar recommendations for wrestling, suggesting that bacterial diseases be treated with oral antibiotics for 48 hours and that no draining, oozing, or moist lesions are present [17]. Residual lesions should be covered, but unless also meeting the previous criteria, such coverage is not sufficient to return to play. There are no concrete guidelines for return to play in most other sports for these infections, but it is recommended that the rules for wrestling should be used for any contact or collision sport. Sports with shared equipment or facility use such as gymnastics or aquatic sports should also follow these guidelines to prevent spread of the disease. Noncontact sports and sports without shared equipment such as cross-country running should be judged on a case-by-case basis.

Table 2
Recommended antibiotic guidelines for non–methicillin-resistant *Staphylococcus aureus* bacterial dermatoses

Dermatosis	Antibiotic regimen[a]	Comments
Impetigo	Local: topical mupirocin tid × 10 d Widespread: add cephalexin 500 mg po qid × 7 d or azithromycin 500 mg po × 1 d, then 250 mg po × 4 d	
Staphylococcus folliculitis	Cephalexin 500 mg po qid × 7 d, or erythromycin 500 mg po qid × 7 d or azithromycin 500 mg po × 1 d, then 250 mg po × 4 d	
Pseudofolliculitis barbae	No antibiotics warranted unless superinfected, then treat as *Staphylococcus* folliculitis	See text for interventions
Pseudomonas folliculitis	Self-limiting, no antibiotics usually warranted If recalcitrant, consider ciprofloxacin 500 mg po bid × 7 d	
Cellulitis	Cephalexin 500 mg po qid × 7 d or erythromycin 500 mg po qid × 7 d	
Furuncles/abscesses	Incision and drainage is definitive treatment, often need to treat for cellulitis as above Strongly consider MRSA treatment empirically	
Pitted keratolysis	Topical 1% clindamycin bid × 10–14 d or topical 2% erythromycin bid × 10–14 d	Ensure drying measures and good hygiene
Erythrasma	Mild: topical 1% clindamycin bid × 7–10 d or topical 2% erythromycin bid × 7–10 d Severe: consider adding erythromycin 250 mg po qid × 5–14 d or clarithromycin 1 g po × 1 dose or tetracycline 250 po qid × 14 d	Consider fungal coinfection

[a]Adult doses given.

Table 3
Wrestling return-to-play guidelines for bacterial dermatoses

Dermatosis	National Collegiate Athletic Association Guidelines	National Federation of High Schools Guidelines
Impetigo, *Staphylococcus* folliculitis, furuncles, abscesses, erisypelas, cellulites	No new lesions for 48 h	Oral antibiotics for 48 h
	Completed 72 h of oral antibiotics No moist, exudative, or draining lesions	No drainage, oozing, or moist lesions
Pseudomonas folliculitis	Not passed skin to skin	Not passed skin to skin
Pitted keratolysis	No guidelines listed	No guidelines listed
Erythrasma	No guidelines listed, would treat as other bacterial infections above	No guidelines listed, would treat as other bacterial infections above

FOLLICULITIS
Description and Diagnosis
Folliculitis is a broad term referring to inflammation of the superficial portion of hair follicles usually occurring as small pustules on an erythematous base [18]. Three types of folliculitis are discussed in this section: *Staphylococcus* folliculitis, pseudofolliculitis barbae ("razor bumps"), and *Pseudomonas* folliculitis ("hot tub folliculitis"). Although similar in appearance, patient history and distribution patterns of the lesions are usually sufficient for making the diagnosis and rendering appropriate treatment. If cultures are needed, swabbing is usually ineffective, so an entire lesion should be shaved off superficially and placed on culture media [10].

Staphylococcus folliculitis is the most common of the three forms discussed here. It can occur on any portion of the body but is most often found under thigh pads or other occlusive barriers. Lesions may be slightly pruritic to mildly painful [14]. Systemic symptoms of fevers, chills, or malaise can occur if lesions are widespread. Superficial infections without abscesses or fluctuance are usually methicillin sensitive, although MRSA infections should be suspected if not responding to antibiotics traditionally effective against gram-positive organisms.

Pseudomonas folliculitis, or hot tub folliculitis, occurs most frequently from contact with poorly cleaned hot tubs or whirlpools but can also be from shared sponges or cleaning products. Although lesions tend to be pruritic, urticarial, and erythematous and most frequently occur as clustered lesions on occluded areas under bathing suits (Fig. 2) [19], localized reactions (such as on feet or hands) have occurred due to contaminated water [20].

Pseudofolliculitis barbae is not truly a bacterial infection, being due to a foreign body reaction to ingrown hairs, but there is often bacterial

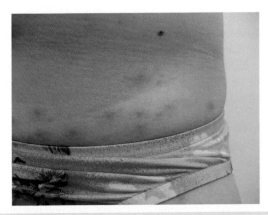

Fig. 2. *Pseudomonas* (hot tub) folliculitis. (*Courtesy of* Daniel L. Stulberg, MD, Denver, CO.)

superinfection at the site [10]. Lesions appear similar to those of staphylococcal origin, although with less inflammation present. The back of the neck is most commonly affected, but this entity can occur on any shaved surface of skin.

Differential Diagnosis

The three types of folliculitis discussed may be distinguished by the descriptions in the previous paragraphs, but a variety of other illnesses may present with similar lesions. These illnesses include dermatophyte infections, cutaneous candidiasis, acne vulgaris, acne mechanica, steroid-induced acne, and keratosis pilaris.

Treatment and Return to Play

Oral antibiotics are the treatment of choice for MSSA infections (see Table 2). Regimens include cephalexin (500 mg) orally four times a day for 7 days, erythromycin (500 mg) orally four times a day for 7 days, or azithromycin (500 mg) orally for 1 day, then 250 mg orally for 4 days. Concomitant use of topical antibacterial soaps may help prevent recurrence. Known carriers of MRSA or those at high risk warrant treatment with doxycycline or trimethoprim/sulfamethoxazole as described in Table 1. *Pseudomonas* folliculitis is self-limiting in 5 to 7 days and does not usually respond to antibiotics, although some recommend quinolone therapy (eg, ciprofloxacin, 500 mg orally twice daily for 7 days) for recalcitrant cases [11]. Pseudofolliculitis barbae is often the most difficult folliculitis to treat and involves stopping shaving the affected areas, manually releasing entrapped hairs with a sterile needle, and consideration of a short course (5–7 days) of systemic MSSA-effective antibiotics for persistent lesions [10].

Return-to-play criteria for *Staphylococcus* folliculitis is the same as for other bacterial dermatoses and ranges from 48 to 72 hours of systemic antibiotics with no moist, oozing, or exudative lesions and no new lesions in 48 hours (see Table 3). Due to the high rates of concomitant infection, those who have pseudofolliculitis barbae should follow the same protocol. *Pseudomonas* folliculitis is not passed by way of skin-to-skin contact [10], but if any ambiguity is present as to the diagnosis, the return-to-play guidelines for staphylococcal lesions should be followed. It is essential to follow proper cleaning techniques of any whirlpool or hot tub suspected of contamination with *Pseudomonas* because large outbreaks have been known to occur from a single source.

FURUNCLES AND ABSCESSES
Description and Diagnosis
Furuncles, abscesses, and carbuncles present as painful, erythematous, fluctuant, circumscribed masses. Early lesions may resemble erysipelas or cellulitis but usually progress rapidly. Hyperhidrosis and occlusion are risk factors for developing furunculosis. Systemic symptoms are notably absent, although surrounding cellulitis can occur [11]. Most common sites are groin, axilla, and posterior thighs due to the presence of friction [15], but lesions may also occur on the ear or face. *Staphylococcus aureus* is the most common pathogen, but in the perianal region, gram-negative pathogens may be causative [10].

Differential Diagnosis
Other skin conditions can mimic bacterial abscesses, including epidermal cysts, hidradenitis suppurativa, and cystic acne. Early lesions may resemble cellulitis, trauma, or erysipelas, but progression to fluctuance distinguishes enclosed lesions from diffuse ones.

Treatment and Return to Play
Treatment of enclosed lesions can be done with warm compresses and antibiotics, but definitive treatment is usually accomplished only by incision and drainage. Larger or loculated lesions may need a draining wick inserted. Usually, no systemic antibiotics are warranted in an immunocompetent host, but if cellulitis is present, antibiotics should be administered in dosing regimens described under the "Cellulitis and erysipelas" section and with strong consideration of treating for MRSA.

Despite the fact that definitive treatment may not require systemic antibiotics, treatment may facilitate return to play by limiting transmission in contact and collision sports. Return-to-play guidelines are the same as those discussed earlier and include appropriate systemic antibiotics for 48 to 72 hours, no new lesions for 48 hours, and no actively draining lesions at time of play (see Table 3).

CELLULITIS AND ERYSIPELAS
Description and Diagnosis
The triad of erythema, edema, and pain characterizes these infections [10,11,15]. Erysipelas refers to only superficial infection of the skin, with well-demarcated borders and often lymphangitis. Cellulitis, however, implies subcutaneous involvement. Fever and lymphadenopathy may be present, particularly with extensive disease. Skin trauma or chronic damage are

predisposing factors but they may or may not be present. Many different pathogens can cause infection, including gram-negative pathogens and atypical bacteria, but in the athletic population, group A *Streptococcus* and *Staphylococcus* species are by far the most common [18].

Culture of lesions at the leading edge used to be routine but is no longer recommended [15]. If systemic symptoms are severe, then blood cultures are warranted, but in most cases, the diagnosis is made clinically and the treatment is initiated empirically.

Differential diagnosis
Trauma or superficial burns may mimic these infections, but usually the clinical triad described previously usually secures the diagnosis.

Treatment and Return to Play
Treatment of these infections should be driven not only by the prevalence of MRSA in the community but also by the degree of involvement. A small area of peripheral (arm or leg) infection may be treated with a first-generation cephalosporin (eg, cephalexin, 500 mg orally four times daily for 7–10 days) or macrolide (eg, erythromycin, 500 mg four times daily for 7–10 days) if close follow-up is provided and the patient can be changed to MRSA-appropriate antibiotics if lesions are extending. Any sensitive areas (groin, hands, and so forth) in a community with known MRSA should be treated with doxycyclin (100 mg) orally twice a day or trimethoprim/sulfamethoxazole DS orally twice a day for 10 to 14 days with close observation. Extensive cellulitis or patients who have systemic symptoms may warrant hospitalization for intravenous antibiotics. Although rare, providers should also observe for synovitis or septic joints underlying cellulitic areas.

Return to play is discussed previously (see Table 3) and involves treatment for 48 to 72 hours with systemic antibiotics. For cellulitis in particular, it bears mention that no patient should return to play with a fever or other systemic symptoms.

PITTED KERATOLYSIS
Description and Diagnosis
Pitted keratolysis, also called "sweaty sock syndrome," is a bacterial infection affecting the feet. Originally recognized in bare-footed people in tropical regions, it is now recognized to have a global distribution and to commonly affect athletes. The most common clinical manifestation is hyperhydrosis of the skin, usually accompanied by malodor and sliminess of the skin. Characteristic pitting of the soles is a key finding in distinguishing the infection (Fig. 3) [10,14]. Lesions are most often found on the pressure-bearing aspects of the sole of the feet and, although they have been reported, they are rare elsewhere on the foot [21].

Multiple bacteria have been implicated in pitted keratolysis, including *Dermatophilius* and *Micrococcus* [10]. These bacteria can excrete keratinase, which degrades the skin and causes the characteristic pitting. If presentation and

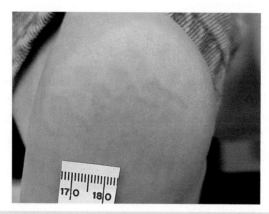

Fig. 3. Characteristic pitting of pitted keratolysis. (*Courtesy of* Daniel L. Stulberg, MD, Denver, CO.)

history are characteristic of the diagnosis, there is usually no need for laboratory confirmation or bacterial cultures. If confirmation is needed, the most reliable method is to shave specimens of keratin and examine them microscopically with staining.

Differential Diagnosis

The differential diagnosis of pitted keratolysis includes fungal infections (tinea pedis) and mechanical/environmental injury (trench foot). The pitting and distribution pattern of lesions that occurs almost exclusively on weight-bearing areas, however, distinguishes this disease from tinea pedis and trench foot.

Treatment and Return to Play

Treatment starts by modifying environmental conditions, particularly frequent drying and the use of moisture-wicking synthetic socks. Aluminum chloride (Drysol) or a 10% formaldehyde solution as an antiperspirant may also be effective [18]. Antibiotic therapy with topical 2% erythromycin or 1% clindamycin (applied twice daily for duration of lesions) is also highly effective [10,22]. There are no restrictions on return to play for athlete who have pitted keratolysis.

ERYTHRASMA

Description and Diagnosis

Erythrasma is characterized by patchy, erythematous, irregular plaques usually affecting the interdigital spaces of the feet. Although it often accompanies inflammatory conditions, erythrasma in and of itself does not tend to be significantly pruritic or irritating. Caused by a *Corynebacterium*, it is the most common bacterial infection of the foot, although it can also occur in any moist environment such as the axilla, groin, or intergluteal areas (Fig. 4) [23]. Obesity,

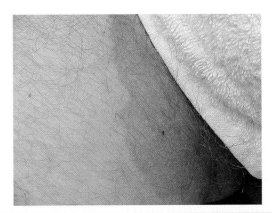

Fig. 4. Erythrasma in groin under regular light. (*Courtesy of* Daniel L. Stulberg, MD, Denver, CO.)

hyperhidrosis, diabetes, immunocompromisation, and poor hygiene are risk factors for acquiring the disease.

Diagnosis of the lesions can be made by the characteristic coral-red fluorescing of lesions under a Wood's light examination (Fig. 5) [10]. Gram stain may show gram-positive rod-shaped organisms. Bacterial cultures are also possible but are not always as reliable or practical [10].

Differential Diagnosis

Any inflammatory condition of intertriginous areas can be considered in the differential for erythrasma. This includes dermatophytosis, psoriasis, or candidiasis. To complicate matters, there are often coexisting fungal infections with

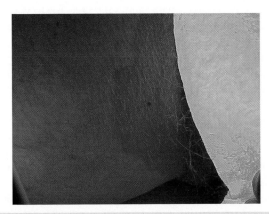

Fig. 5. Coral-red appearance of erythrasma in groin under fluorescent (Wood's) light. (*Courtesy of* Daniel L. Stulberg, MD, Denver, CO.)

bacterial erythrasma. Some studies have shown, for example, that up to 30% of patients affected by erythrasma also have concomitant *Candida* infection [23]. Likewise, erythrasma should be considered in any player not improving from treatment of a "fungal infection" with topical antifungal therapy.

Treatment and Return to Play

Topical 2% erythromycin or 1% clindamycin applied twice daily for 14 days has been found to be fairly effective, as has topical 2% miconozole cream applied twice daily for 14 days. Ketoconazole is not an effective agent [10]. Most investigators favor a systemic or combined systemic/topical approach (see Table 2). Regimens include erythromycin (250 mg) four times a day for 5 days [10] to 14 days [23]. Clarithromycin (1 g) in a single dose is easier, better tolerated, and has similar clinical efficacy [10,23]. Tetracycline (250 mg) four times a day for 14 days is also a reasonable therapy [23]. There is also some new evidence that red-light photodynamic treatment may also be effective [24], although lesions may not be treated to cure using this approach.

There are no return-to-play guidelines recommended for erythrasma, but the disease has been shown to be contagious among teams and military recruits [23]; therefore, the authors recommend treatment for 48 to 72 hours before return to contact situations (see Table 3). It is a reasonable approach to treat even asymptomatic players and to isolate them from communal showers until lesions are clear.

OTHER UNUSUAL DERMATOSES

Mycobacterium Infections

Nontuberculous *Mycobacterium* infections are rare and may manifest as a systemic rather than a cutaneous infection, but one skin entity bears mention. *Mycobacterium marinum* can cause granulomatous infections of the skin, often called "swimming pool granuloma." This infection can occur in fishermen or swimmers who have contact with contaminated fresh water or saltwater swimming areas. Incubation ranges from several days to several weeks, and the infection usually presents as a nonhealing nodular lymphangitis, usually at a site of minor trauma [10]. Lesions may cause tenosynovitis if located over superficial tendons (eg, on the hands) and may cause ulcerated lesions. Treatment is minocycline (100 mg) twice daily for 3 months to 1 year [25].

Necrotizing Fasciitis

Necrotizing fasciitis is an extremely rare entity that presents as a simple cellulitis but rapidly progresses over 6 to 36 hours to sepsis and, frequently, death. Caused most frequently by group A *Streptococcus* but occasionally by anaerobes, this infection should be suspected in any athlete who has rapidly progressive symptoms, pain out of proportion to the appearance of infection, exquisitely tender lesions, or any signs or symptoms of sepsis. Treatment is immediate hospitalization for systemic broad-spectrum antibiotics and surgical debridement. Mortality is approximately 25% [10].

CONSIDERATIONS IN PREVENTION OF BACTERIAL DERMATOSES

There are many common themes in the previous discussion of disease entities. Moist environments, player hygiene, close conditions in locker or team rooms, and player's immune systems factor into the frequency and severity of bacterial infection [26]. Team physicians can play an active role in prevention of these diseases not only by following return-to-play guidelines but also by teaching coaches, trainers, and players to follow some simple guidelines:

Proper nutrition and rest to maintain athlete immune systems
Appropriate personal hygiene techniques, including minimization of contact, frequent hand-washing, occlusion of lesions, wearing sandals in the shower, and notification of the trainer for any lesions
No sharing of towels or protective gear among team members
Ensuring immunizations are up to date

Appropriate standards of disinfection should also be followed for equipment, pads, and mats. Inadequate disinfection or incomplete treatment of carriers or infected athletes often ensures a cycle of recurring infection among a team or institution [27].

SUMMARY

Bacterial infections, including MRSA infections, are common in the athletic setting. Taking proper preventative measures, rapidly recognizing and treating infections, and following conservative return-to-play guidelines ensure that the risk to athletes is minimized.

References

[1] Salgado CD, Farr BM, Calfee DP. Community acquired methicillin-resistant *Staphylococcus aureus*: a meta-analysis of prevalence and risk factors. Clin Infect Dis 2003;36:131–9.
[2] Palavecino E. Community-acquired methicillin-resistant *Staphylococcus aureus* infections. Clin Lab Med 2004;24(2):403–18.
[3] Kuehnert MJ, Kruszon-Moran D, Hill HA, et al. Prevalence of *Staphylococcus aureus* nasal colonization in the United States, 2001–2002. J Infect Dis 2006;193(2):172–9.
[4] Cohen PR, Kurzrock R. Community-acquired methicillin-resistant *Staphylococcus aureus* skin infection: an emerging clinical problem. Clin Infect Dis 2005;4:100–7.
[5] Kazakova SV, Hageman JC, Matava M, et al. A clone of methicillin-resistant *Staphylococcus aureus* among professional football players. N Engl J Med 2005;352(5):468–75.
[6] Begier EM, Frenette K, Barrett NL, et al. A high-morbidity outbreak of methicillin-resistant *Staphylococcus aureus* among players on a college football team, facilitated by cosmetic body shaving and turf burns. Clin Infect Dis 2004;39(10):1446–53.
[7] Lindenmayer JM, Schoenfeld S, O'Grady R, et al. Methicillin-resistant *Staphylococcus aureus* in a high school wrestling team and the surrounding community. Arch Intern Med 1998;158:895–9.
[8] Romano R, Lu D, Holtom P. Outbreaks of community acquired methicillin resistant *Staphylococcus aureus* skin infections among a collegiate football team. J Athl Train 2006;4(5):141–5.
[9] Loeb M, Main C, Walker-Dilks C, et al. Antimicrobial drugs for treating methicillin-resistant staphylococcus aureus. Cochrane Database Syst Rev 2003;(4):CD003340.

[10] Habif T. Clinical dermatology. 4th edition. Philadelphia: Mosby; 2004. p. 264–306.

[11] O'Dell ML. Skin and wound infections: an overview. Am Fam Physician 1998;57(10): 2424–32.

[12] Ludlam H, Cookson B. Scrum kidney: epidemic pyoderma caused by a nephritogenic *Streptococcus pyogenes* in a rugby team. Lancet 1986;2(8502):331–3.

[13] Taylor JS. Cochrane for clinicians—interventions for impetigo. Am Fam Physician 2004;70(9):1680–1.

[14] Adams BB. Dermatologic disorders of the athlete. Sports Med 2002;32(5):309–21.

[15] Cordoro KM, Ganz JE. Training room management of medical conditions: sports dermatology. Clin Sports Med 2005;24:565–98.

[16] Bubb RB. 2006 NCAA wrestling rules and interpretations. Indianapolis (IN): National Collegiate Athletic Association; 2006.

[17] National Federation of High Schools, Sports Medicine Advisory Committee. Physician release for wrestlers to participate with skin lesion(s). Available at: www.nfhs.org. Accessed October 18, 2006.

[18] Adams BB. Sports dermatology. Dermatol Nurs 2001;13(5):347–63.

[19] Freiman A, Barankin B, Elpern D. Sports dermatology part 2: swimming and other aquatic sports. CMAJ 2004;171(11):1339–41.

[20] Green JJ. Localized whirlpool folliculitis in a football player. Cutis 2000;65(6):359–62.

[21] Takama H, Tamada Y, Yano K, et al. Pitted keratolysis: clinical manifestations in 53 cases. Br J Dermatol 1997;137(2):282–5.

[22] Pharis DB, Teller C, Wolf JE Jr. Cutaneous manifestations of sports participation. J Am Acad Dermatol 1997;36(3 Pt 1):448–59.

[23] Holdiness MR. Management of cutaneous erythrasma. Drugs 2002;62(8):1131–41.

[24] Darras-Vercambre S, Carpentier O, Vincent P, et al. Photodynamic action of red light for treatment of erythrasma. Photodermatol Photoimmunol Photomed 2006;22(3):153–6.

[25] Bartralot R, Garcia-Patos V, Sitjas D, et al. Clinical patterns of cutaneous nontuberculous mycobacterial infections. Br J Dermatol 2005;152(4):727–34.

[26] Howe WB. Preventing infectious disease in sports. Phys Sports Med 2003;31(2):23–9.

[27] Center for Disease Control (CDC). Methicillin-resistant *Staphylococcus aureus* infections among competitive sports participants—Colorado, Indiana, Pennsylvania, and Los Angeles County, 2000–2003. MMWR Morb Mortal Wkly Rep 2003;52(33):793–5. Available at: www.cdc.gov/mmwr . Accessed October 18, 2006.

Clin Sports Med 26 (2007) 397–411

CLINICS IN SPORTS MEDICINE

ELSEVIER
SAUNDERS

Cutaneous Fungal and Viral Infections in Athletes

Michael D. Pleacher, MD[a],*, William W. Dexter, MD, FACSM[b,c]

[a]McKay-Dee Sports Medicine, 4403 Harrison Blvd., Suite 2440, Ogden, UT 84403, USA
[b]Sports Medicine Program, Maine Medical Center, 272 Congress Street, Portland, ME 04101, USA
[c]Family Practice Residency Program, Maine Medical Center, 272 Congress Street, Portland, ME 04101, USA

Athletes may be affected by a variety of cutaneous fungal and viral infections. Participation in athletic activities with active skin infections may lead to outbreaks of disease among teammates and competitors. Such outbreaks have been sufficiently common as to lead to the widespread use of medical terms such as tinea gladiatorum and herpes gladiatorum to identify fungal and viral infections spread during athletic activity. Physicians caring for athletes must be familiar with the clinical presentations of common fungal and viral infections. The physician should also be facile with diagnostic tests and appropriate treatment regimens for these infections. Adverse drug reactions, particularly with oral antifungal and antiviral agents, are common and should be recognizable to the treating physician. The team physician must also be aware of the return-to-play regulations enforced by the various sport governing bodies. A thorough knowledge of the common cutaneous fungal and viral infections allows the physician to accurately diagnose and treat these conditions.

CUTANEOUS FUNGAL INFECTIONS: GENERAL CONSIDERATIONS

Pathophysiology

Superficial cutaneous fungal infections are caused by dermatophytes, which are a diverse group of organisms that grow in soil, on humans, and on animals [1]. There are three major genera of dermatophytes: *Trychophyton, Microsporum,* and *Epidermophyton.* Transmission of dermatophytes may occur by direct person-to-person contact, contact with fomites, animal-to-human contact, or directly from the soil [2]. Infection of the skin with dermatophytes is limited to the stratum corneum. The body responds to this infection by increasing proliferation of the basal cell layer, which results in epidermal thickening and the formation of scale on the lesion [3].

*Corresponding author. E-mail address: mike.pleacher@intermountainmail.org (M.D. Pleacher).

0278-5919/07/$ – see front matter
doi:10.1016/j.csm.2007.04.004

Dermatophyte infection results in a variety of clinical manifestations. Infection of the skin and hair on the scalp is termed tinea capitis. Infections occurring on the body are termed tinea corporis, commonly called ringworm. Infections in the groin (commonly called jock-itch) are named tinea cruris. Fungal infections of the feet are termed tinea pedis, or athlete's foot. Dermatophytes can also infect the toenails, a condition termed onychomycosis [2].

Epidemiology

Between 10% and 20% of the population worldwide is estimated to be infected with a dermatophyte. The most common clinical manifestation of dermatophyte infection is tinea pedis, occurring in up to 70% of adults worldwide over a lifetime [4]. Dermatophyte infection appears to be more common among persons of African American and Asian heritage [5].

Clinical Presentation

Cutaneous fungal infections present with various clinical appearances. An annular patch of hair loss often characterizes tinea capitis, with an underlying gray, hyperkeratotic plaque on the scalp [2]. The lesions of tinea corporis are well-defined erythematous plaques, often with a raised border and central clearing as demonstrated in Fig. 1. Flaking and pruritis may also be present. The head, neck, trunk, and upper extremities are the most common sites of infection for athletes who have tinea corporis [6]. Tinea cruris is characterized by the development of large, erythematous, well-demarcated scaling plaques in the pubic area, inguinal folds, and medial thighs [2]. Tinea pedis has a variety of presentations, including the interdigital type, moccasin type, and bullous type. Interdigital tinea pedis is characterized by macerated skin with fissure formation in the web space between toes. The skin is often red and weeping. Moccasin-type tinea pedis, as demonstrated in Fig. 2, presents as a hyperkeratotic erythematous plaque on the sole and sides of the foot. Bullous-type tinea pedis is characterized by the development of vesicles or bullae filled with clear fluid [2].

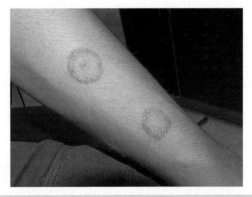

Fig. 1. Tinea corporis (ringworm). (*Courtesy of* Peg Cyr, MD, Portland, ME.)

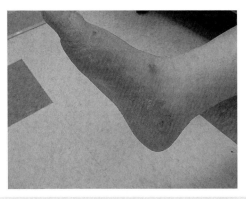

Fig. 2. Moccasin-type tinea pedis. (*Courtesy of* Peg Cyr, MD, Portland, ME.)

Diagnosis

Diagnosis of cutaneous fungal infections is made clinically based on the location and characteristic appearance of the lesions. The diagnosis can be confirmed with direct microscopy of a potassium hydroxide (KOH) preparation or fungal culture. To create the KOH preparation, the examiner removes scale from the leading edge of the plaque and then places the scale on a microscope slide. A coverslip is applied and a 5% to 20% solution of KOH is added. The slide may be heated briefly before examination under a light microscope. A positive KOH preparation reveals septated hyphae on the slide. Fungal culture can be performed, particularly when the lesions are suspicious for fungal infection but the KOH preparation is negative. Sabouraud dextrose agar should be used for the fungal culture [2].

Differential Diagnosis

Tinea capitis, with its annular patch of alopecia, may be mistaken for other conditions causing alopecia, including alopecia areata and trichotillomania; however, these alternate causes of alopecia typically lack the gray scaly appearance common in tinea capitis. Tinea corporis and tinea cruris may be mistaken for impetigo, psoriasis, lichen planus, seborrheic dermatitis, pityriasis rosea, and secondary or tertiary syphilis. A positive KOH preparation or fungal culture helps to differentiate these various conditions. Erythrasma, a chronic *Corynebacterium* infection, may mimic tinea cruris; however, erythrasma fluoresces a coral-red color when examined under Wood's light. An acceptable treatment for erythrasma is a 2-week course of erythromycin (250 mg) taken four times daily [7].

Treatment

Superficial cutaneous fungal infections may be treated with topical or oral medications. The topical agents include the imidazoles, allylamines, and naphthiomates. Oral agents include griseofulvin and oral preparations of allylamines and imidazoles. The topical agents are generally well tolerated, but the oral agents can have significant side effects. The fungicidal drugs, such as the allylamines, are favored over the fungistatic imidazoles and griseofulvin. Fungicidal medications require shorter courses of therapy and are recommended over the fungistatic drugs in treating athletes. A summary of various treatment regimens for cutaneous fungal infections appears in Table 1.

The treatment of tinea capitis requires an oral agent. In the United States, the only Food and Drug Administration (FDA)-approved oral agent for tinea capitis is griseofulvin. Adult doses of griseofulvin range from 15 to 25 mg/kg daily for a total of 6 to 12 weeks of therapy [8]. Although no other oral agent has an FDA indication for treatment of tinea capitis, agents such as ketoconazole, itraconazole, and fluconazole can be used to successfully treat this infection. Treatment regimens are generally shorter with the oral azole agents. Adults can be successfully treated with itraconazole (200 mg daily for 2–4 weeks), fluconazole (6 mg/kg daily for 3–6 weeks), or ketoconazole (200 mg daily for 2–4 weeks) [8,9].

Treatment of noninflammatory tinea corporis and tinea cruris is typically initiated with topical medications. Oral therapy is reserved for patients who have extensive or disabling disease at presentation, patients who are immunosuppressed, or patients who have failed topical therapy [4]. Topical terbinafine, a fungicidal allylamine, is available in a 1% cream that is applied one

Table 1
Summary of treatment regimens for tinea capitis, tinea corporis, tinea cruris, and tinea pedis

Condition	Agent	Dose, frequency	Duration of treatment
Tinea capitis	Griseofulvin	15–25 mg/kg, qd	6–12 wk
	Itraconazole	200 mg, qd	2–4 wk
	Fluconazole	6 mg/kg, qd	3–6 wk
	Ketoconazole	200 mg, qd	2–4 wk
Tinea corporis and tinea cruris	Terbinafine 1% cream	Topical, qd–bid	2–4 wk
	Ketoconazole 2% cream	Topical, qd	2–4 wk
	Clotrimazole 1% cream	Topical, qd	2–4 wk
	Griseofulvin	500 mg orally, qd	2–4 wk
	Itraconazole	100 mg orally, qd	2 wk
	Terbinafine	250 mg orally, qd	1 wk
	Fluconazole	150 mg orally, weekly	2–4 wk
Tinea pedis	Ketoconazole 2% cream	Topical, qd	4–6 wk
	Clotrimazole 1% cream	Topical, qd	4–6 wk

to two times daily for 2 to 4 weeks. A 1-week course of terbinafine 1% cream has been shown to be effective in 84% of cases [10]. Ketoconazole 2% cream is typically applied once daily for 2 to 4 weeks. A study of once-daily application of ketoconazole 2% cream demonstrated improvement in symptoms among most patients treated for 4 weeks, with a relapse rate of 7.2% 4 weeks after cessation of therapy [11]. Clotrimazole is available in cream, lotion, and solution formulations and is generally applied daily for 2 to 4 weeks.

Cases of tinea corporis and tinea cruris that fail topical therapy require systemic treatment. Available oral treatments include griseofulvin, itraconazole, terbinafine, and fluconazole. Griseofulvin has been shown to be effective at doses of 500 mg daily for 2 to 4 weeks; however, a significant number of patients, as many as 12.5% in one study, developed adverse drug reactions [12]. Griseofulvin may induce paresthesias, it may elevate serum transaminases, and it may induce leukopenia. Far more common are the mild side effects including headache, rash, and photosensitivity. Physicians caring for athletes treated with griseofulvin must counsel the athlete about these potential adverse effects. Athletes competing outdoors must be aware of the photosensitivity and use sun block while on griseofulvin. Itraconazole has been shown to be effective in the treatment of tinea corporis and tinea cruris. Doses of 100 mg taken daily for 2 weeks results in clinical cure or improvement in 96% of patients. Side effects are common (20% of patients in one study) but are generally mild and include headache, dyspepsia, and flatulence [13]. Oral terbinafine (250 mg taken daily for 1 week) has also proved effective in the treatment of tinea corporis and tinea cruris. This regimen resulted in mycologic cure in 100% of patients and was well tolerated, with no adverse events reported [14]. Fluconazole has also been examined in tinea corporis and tinea cruris. Patients treated with 150 mg fluconazole once weekly for 2 to 4 weeks had significant improvement in symptom scores, with mycologic cure documented in over 80% of patients. Side effects were rare and generally limited to mild gastrointestinal upset [15].

Treatment of tinea pedis may be undertaken with topical or oral medications. Mild cases of tinea pedis often respond favorably to topical therapy, whereas moderate, severe, or chronic cases of tinea pedis may require oral therapy. Inflammatory cases of tinea pedis may require the addition of a topical steroid to improve symptoms. A Cochrane Database Systematic Review examining the topical allylamines naftifine and terbinafine found that both medications were equally effective in treating tinea pedis compared with placebo. This same systematic review found that treatment of tinea pedis with a topical azole for 4 to 6 weeks was significantly more effective in producing a mycologic cure compared with placebo. The azoles were proven superior to allylamines in curing tinea pedis [16]. A recent Cochrane Database Systematic Review revealed that terbinafine taken orally was somewhat more effective in inducing cure compared with griseofulvin. Cure rates were comparable among oral terbinafine, fluconazole, itraconazole, and ketoconazole [17].

CUTANEOUS FUNGAL INFECTIONS: CONSIDERATIONS SPECIFIC TO ATHLETES

Tinea Gladiatorum

Tinea gladiatorum is a term used to describe fungal infections of the skin or scalp among athletes. The causative organisms for outbreaks of tinea gladiatorum are generally species within the *Trychophyton* genus. These infections often cluster among teammates and competitors. The warm, moist environment coupled with occlusive clothing and equipment facilitate the development of cutaneous fungal infections. Close skin-to-skin contact among athletes facilitates the direct person-to-person transmission of the fungi. Wrestling equipment including the mats and headgear may be fomites, leading to transmission of the dermatophyte [6]. One recent study, however, indicated that no dermatophytes were isolated from the wrestling equipment in an area with a widespread dermatophyte outbreak [18].

Among the general population, *T tonsurans* is the most common causative agent for tinea capitis. *T rubrum* is the most commonly isolated pathogen in cases of tinea corporis in the general population, with *T tonsurans* a distant second [19]. Among athletes, particularly wrestlers, *T tonsurans* is the most commonly implicated pathogen causing tinea gladiatorum [6]. Stiller and colleagues [20] reported on one of the earliest outbreaks of tinea gladiatorum in the United States. These investigators reported on five cases of *T tonsurans* infection among high school and collegiate wrestlers in northern New York. Similar epidemics have occurred in Alaska, Sweden, and Lanzarote, with 21, 19, and 45 wrestlers infected with *T tonsurans*, respectively [21–23]. In the Alaskan study, this number represented a 75% prevalence rate [21]. Forty-four percent of the wrestlers examined in Lanzarote were infected [23]. The prevalence of tinea gladiatorum among wrestlers in another study in Ohio was lower (24%) [24]. A survey of high schools in Pennsylvania revealed that over 84% of responding schools had at least one wrestler diagnosed with tinea gladiatorum during the 1998 to 1999 wrestling season [25].

The diagnosis of tinea gladiatorum is made as described earlier. The team physician and athletic training staff should be vigilant in screening athletes, particularly once an outbreak has been identified. Treatment of wrestlers who have tinea gladiatorum does not differ significantly from general treatment of patients who have tinea corporis or tinea cruris, although generally it is recommended that a fungicidal medication be used when possible. A small prospective study comparing clotrimazole 1% cream with oral fluconazole (200 mg weekly) in the treatment of tinea gladiatorum found no statistically significant differences in symptom reduction and mycologic cure rates between the two regimens [26]. A larger blinded, placebo-controlled study examined the efficacy of fluconazole in the prevention of tinea gladiatorum. There was a significantly lower incidence of infection (6% versus 22%) among wrestlers treated with fluconazole (100 mg weekly) compared with those treated with weekly placebo [27]. The findings of the preventative study, however, have not been replicated, and this practice has not been universally adopted.

Team physicians will be asked to render an opinion on when it is safe for a wrestler who has tinea gladiatorum to return to competition. Early recommendations by Beller and Gessner [21] were to disqualify wrestlers until lesions had been treated with 10 days of topical therapy or 15 days of oral therapy and were showing signs of improvement. The National Collegiate Athletic Association (NCAA) regulations (Table 2) require a wrestler to be disqualified from practice or competition until a minimum of 72 hours of topical fungicidal treatment has been completed. Athletes who have scalp lesions must be treated with a minimum of 2 weeks of oral therapy before returning to competition. Lesions must be covered with a gas-permeable dressing for competition. Examples of gas-permeable dressings include Tegaderm (3M, St Paul, MN), Bioclusive (Ethicon, Somerville, NJ), and Opsite (Smith & Nephew Wound Management, Largo, FL) dressings. Written documentation outlining the diagnosis, treatment, and dates of treatment are required [28]. The National Federation of State High School Associations (NFHS) recommends the use of a standardized form to communicate information from physicians to coaches regarding skin

Table 2
Summary of return-to-play guidelines for fungal and viral infections in athletes

Condition	NCAA guidelines	NFHS recommendations
Tinea capitis	Minimum 2 wk of oral griseofulvin before return to play	Minimum 2 wk of oral griseofulvin before return to play
Tinea corporis	Minimum 72 h of a topical fungicide Lesions must be covered with a gas-permeable membrane	Oral or topical treatment for 7 d Written release from team physician to coach
Primary herpes gladiatorum	Free of systemic symptoms for 72 h No new lesions for at least 72 h Oral antiviral treatment for at least 120 h	120 h of oral antiviral treatment No new lesions appearing while on antiviral treatment
Reactivation herpes gladiatorum	No moist lesions 120 h of oral antiviral treatment	120 h of oral antiviral treatment No new lesions appearing while on antiviral treatment
Molluscum contagiosum	Local lesions may be covered with gas-permeable dressings Extensive lesions must be curetted or removed	Curettage followed by 24 h before return to play
Verrucae vulgaris	Lesions must be adequately covered	No official position

Abbreviation: NFHS, National Federation of State High School Associations.

infections in athletes. The NFHS recommends that athletes who have tinea gladiatorum be treated with oral or topical treatment for 7 days before returning to competition, unless the lesions are on the scalp, in which a minimum of 2 weeks of oral therapy is recommended before returning to play [29].

Tinea Pedis

Tinea pedis occurs commonly in athletes. A large European study revealed that 36.1% of sports-active individuals had evidence of fungal infection of the feet [30]. Swimming pool users have been shown to have a high rate of dermatophyte infection [31]. Marathon runners similarly have a high incidence of active and subclinical tinea pedis [32,33]. The diagnosis and treatment of athletes who have tinea pedis is as described earlier. There are no specific rules guiding return-to-play decisions in athletes who have tinea pedis.

CUTANEOUS VIRAL INFECTIONS IN ATHLETES

Athletes may be infected with a variety of viral agents. Factors such as excessive sweating, occlusive clothing, and close skin-to-skin contact in certain sports increase the risk for athletes of developing viral cutaneous infections. The wear of abrasive shirts has been postulated as another potential contributor to the development of herpetic epidemics among wrestlers [34]. Outbreaks of herpes simplex, herpes zoster, molluscum contagiosum, and verrucae vulgaris (warts) have occurred in various groups of athletes. This following sections focus on herpes simplex, molluscum contagiosum, and warts in athletes.

Herpes Simplex

Pathophysiology

Herpes simplex virus (HSV) can cause primary and recurrent infections in athletes. Herpes simplex type 1 is responsible for most cases of herpes labialis. Urogenital herpes is generally caused by herpes simplex type 2. Transmission is by direct skin-to-skin contact. The incubation period ranges from 2 to 20 days in patients experiencing a primary infection. Reactivation of latent herpetic infection from neural ganglia is often heralded by a tingling or burning sensation before the appearance of any overt skin changes. Reactivation may be triggered by physical or emotional stress, UV radiation, fever, or immunosuppression [2].

Epidemiology

HSV infections may occur among athletes. It has been a sufficiently common occurrence in wrestling to coin the term herpes gladiatorum. In rugby athletes, herpetic infection is termed scrumpox. One of the earliest case reports on HSV infection transmitted among wrestlers was published in the *Journal of the American Medical Association* in 1965 [35]. Subsequently, numerous outbreaks of herpes gladiatorum have been reported in high school and college wrestlers [36–38]. Among high school wrestlers at a summer wrestling camp, 60 of 175 developed HSV lesions. These lesions were most commonly found on the head, extremities, and trunk; however, five wrestlers developed ocular involvement [39,40]. A survey of high school and college wrestlers placed the annual incidence of HSV lesions at 7.6% of college wrestlers and 2.6% of high school wrestlers [41]. Transmission of herpes gladiatorum occurs in a short period of time, with an average of 6.8 days from exposure to development of clinically apparent lesions during one Minnesota high school outbreak. The likelihood of contracting herpes if sparring with an infected partner with an active outbreak was calculated at 32.7% [42].

Clinical presentation and diagnosis

The lesions of HSV appear as a group of vesicles on an erythematous base. The vesicles may then ulcerate, leaving a shallow painful ulcer with surrounding erythema. Herpes lesions are common on the lips (herpes labialis), face, hands (herpetic whitlow), and body. In primary infection, systemic symptoms may develop, including fever, adenopathy, malaise, myalgias, and headache. These systemic symptoms do not usually accompany reactivation infection. Rarely, HSV can infect the eyes, resulting in a severe keratoconjunctivitis. Ophthalmologic referral is recommended in cases of ocular herpes. Healing skin lesions take on a crusted or scabbed appearance before complete resolution, which may take up to 2 to 3 weeks.

Diagnosis of HSV infection is generally made on the characteristic clinical appearance of the lesions. A Tzanck test of fluid obtained from an unroofed vesicle may reveal multinucleated giant cells characteristic of HSV infection. A viral culture may provide definitive diagnosis but takes up to 4 to 5 days for results [2].

Treatment

Treatment strategies for active herpes gladiatorum outbreaks are the same as for genital herpes outbreaks. Commonly used medications include acyclovir, valacyclovir, and famcyclovir. Acyclovir may be given in several different regimens, including 200 mg orally five times daily for 5 days, 400 mg orally three times daily for 5 days, or 800 mg twice daily for 5 days. Valacyclovir is generally given orally as 500 mg twice daily for 5 days. Famcyclovir may be given as a 125-mg dose twice daily for 5 days [43]. A well-designed randomized controlled trial comparing acyclovir and valacyclovir found that there were no significant differences between the two active drugs in terms of the length of the outbreak and time to complete lesion healing. Acyclovir and valacyclovir were shown to be superior to placebo [44]. A study comparing valacyclovir with placebo among wrestlers who had herpes gladiatorum outbreaks found that valacyclovir (500 mg twice daily) resulted in significantly shorter duration of clinically apparent lesions and significantly shorter time to clearance of HSV Polymerase chain reaction (PCR) [45].

Suppressive therapy should be considered in athletes who have had recurrent outbreaks of herpes simplex. Common suppressive regimens include acyclovir (400 mg twice daily), valacyclovir (500–1000 mg once daily), and famcyclovir (250 mg twice daily) [43]. Wrestlers with recurrent herpes gladiatorum were studied to determine the effectiveness of valacyclovir as suppressive therapy in this population. There were significantly fewer outbreaks among athletes taking valacyclovir (500 mg once daily or 1000 mg once daily) compared with athletes taking placebo. Athletes who had a longer (>2 year) history of HSV infection had no outbreaks while on the active medication [46].

Return to play

The NCAA maintains stringent rules regarding wrestlers who have active herpes outbreaks, as shown in Table 2. Wrestlers who have a primary herpes infection must be free of systemic symptoms of disease for 72 hours, must have had no new lesions for a period of 72 hours, must have no moist lesions, and must have been treated with oral antiviral agents for 120 hours before returning to practice or competition. Athletes who have recurrent infections must have no moist lesions and must have been treated for 120 hours with oral antiviral agents before clearance for participation. Questionable cases must be more thoroughly evaluated with a Tzanck test or HSV PCR. Wrestlers should be disqualified until the results of these tests are known [28]. The NFHS echoes the recommendations of the NCAA, by suggesting that wrestlers undergo a minimum of 120 hours of oral antiviral treatment, with no new lesions appearing during that time and with all lesions crusted over [29].

Molluscum Contagiosum

Epidemiology

Molluscum contagiosum is a viral skin infection caused by a member of the Poxviridae family. This disorder is most commonly seen among young children. Adults may contract molluscum contagiosum as a sexually transmitted infection. Athletes, particularly those involved in sports characterized by close skin-to-skin contact with competitors, may also develop and spread molluscum contagiosum. Transmission is by direct skin-to-skin contact with an infected person [2].

Clinical presentation

The lesions of molluscum contagiosum are generally asymptomatic. They appear as round papules or nodules. They are typically skin colored and have a central keratotic plug, resulting in the characteristic "umbilicated" appearance. They are commonly found on the face, neck, and trunk. They may also affect the genitals of adults who have contracted this as a sexually transmitted infection [2].

Treatment

In healthy children and adults who have competent immune systems, these lesions generally resolve in about 6 months. In the immunocompromised host, lesions rarely spontaneously resolve.

Treatment options include curettage, cryosurgery, and electrodesiccation. Nonsurgical options include a variety of topical treatments. Chemical destruction with 0.7% cantharidin is a widely accepted treatment. Cryotherapy involving the use of liquid nitrogen to freeze the lesion is another acceptable treatment. This treatment is commonly available in most primary care offices. The lesion is frozen for a period of 10 to 30 seconds until a halo appears around the lesion. The lesion is allowed to thaw before a second freeze cycle is induced. A single application of a silver nitrate paste has been shown to be effective in up to 89.5% of patients. Seventy percent of the treated patients had clearance of the lesions in 10 to 14 days [47]. Immune modulating therapy is also being studied in cases of molluscum contagiosum. Imiquimod 5% cream applied thrice weekly for 12 weeks was compared with a placebo cream in a recent study involving children who had widespread molluscum contagiosum. The active drug was shown to reduce lesion count by nearly half at 12 weeks compared with placebo [48]. Another study involving older patients who had molluscum contagiosum found that imiquimod 1% cream applied three times a day, 5 consecutive days per week for 4 consecutive weeks was effective in curing 86.3% of the treated lesions–far superior to placebo [49].

Return to play
Athletes may be required to undergo treatment before returning to competition. The NCAA rules for wrestling state that lesions must be curetted or removed before clearance for competition. Localized or solitary lesions may be covered with a gas-permeable dressing and then covered with tape [28]. The NFHS suggests holding a wrestler out of competition for 24 hours following curettage [29].

Verrucae Vulgaris (Warts)
Epidemiology
Common warts are caused by various types of human papillomaviruses (HPV). Genital warts are typically caused by HPV types 6, 11, 16, and 18. HPV types 6 and 11 have little potential for malignant transformation, but types 16 and 18 can lead to malignant change. Warts are transmitted by direct skin-to-skin contact, but infectivity is generally considered low. Immunocompromised hosts have a higher incidence of HPV infections associated with more widespread outbreaks [2].

Clinical presentation and diagnosis
Warts may have numerous clinical presentations. Common warts are firm, small, hyperkeratotic papules that are generally skin-colored. They may appear anywhere on the body but typically affect the hands and fingers. Plantar warts are hyperkeratotic skin-colored plaques found on the plantar surface of the foot. Diagnosis is typically made on the characteristic clinical appearance of the lesions. When the diagnosis is in doubt, excision and dermatopathologic examination may confirm the diagnosis of HPV infection [2].

Treatment
Given enough time, most warts are self-resolving as the virus is recognized and suppressed by the immune system. One early study on the natural history of warts revealed that in children, 40% of warts cleared spontaneously over a 2-year period [50]. Left untreated, however, warts may progress in size and

develop wider distribution as the virus replicates. Warts on the sole of the foot and periungual warts may become painful.

Treatment of warts is similar to treatment of molluscum contagiosum. Surgical removal and destruction of the lesions with cryotherapy are two common methods of treatment. Chemical applications, including salicylic acid preparations or trichloroacetic acid preparations, are also effective in treating warts. Paring down the superficial layers of skin following topical treatments is important so that the cells at the base of the wart where the virus is still actively reproducing are exposed to the next round of treatment. Retreatment is commonly required for warts. Immune modulating agents such as imiquimod may also be effective in treating common warts [2]. Other treatment options include laser therapy, intralesional therapy with bleomycin, topical formulations of 5-fluorouracil, and topical retinoids.

A recent systematic review pooled data from numerous studies looking at local treatment for simple nongenital warts. Salicylic acid was shown to be an effective treatment, with a pooled cure rate of 75% and an odds ratio of 3.91 favoring treatment with salicylic acid. Cryotherapy was shown to be similar in efficacy compared with salicylic acid [51].

Imiquimod 5% cream has been used extensively in the treatment of anogenital warts. It has been successfully used to treat common warts as well. In a group of children who had treatment-resistant warts, imiquimod was used daily for an average of 5 months. Sixteen of 18 patients treated had long-term clearing of their warts [52]. Results in adults treated in a similar manner had less dramatic results, although 27% had complete resolution of their warts, with an additional 49% of those treated having a reduction in number of warts by more than 50% [53]. Another study examined imiquimod in the treatment of warts and found complete clearance in 30% of those treated, with partial clearance in an additional 26% [54].

Definitive data on the most effective strategy for destroying warts is still lacking. The physician and patient must be prepared for a potentially lengthy course of treatment, with widespread treatment failures and recurrences.

Return to play

Athletes involved in sports such as wrestling in which direct skin-to-skin contact is common should have warts treated before competing. The NCAA wrestling rules state that wrestlers must have all lesions "adequately covered" for competition or they will be disqualified [28]. The NFHS has no official position on return to play for athletes who have common cutaneous warts.

SUMMARY

Fungal and viral cutaneous infections are common among athletes, and they can develop quickly into widespread outbreaks. To prevent such outbreaks, the team physician must be familiar with common cutaneous infections, including tinea corporis, tinea capitis, tinea pedis, herpes simplex, molluscum contagiosum, and HPV. Appropriate treatment and management of these infections allows the athlete to safely return to play and safeguards teammates and opponents against the spread of these diseases.

References

[1] Murphy GF, Mihm MC Jr. The skin. In: Cotran RS, Kumar V, Collins T, editors. Robbins pathologic basis of disease. 6th edition. Philadelphia: WB Saunders; 1999. p. 1170–213.

[2] Fitzpatrick TB, Johnson RA, Wolff K, et al, editors. Cutaneous fungal infections . Color atlas and synopsis of clinical dermatology. 3rd edition. New York: McGraw-Hill; 1997. p. 688–733.

[3] Odom R. Pathophysiology of dermatophyte infections. J Am Acad Dermatol 1993;28: S2–7.

[4] Drake LA, Dinehart SM, Farmer ER, et al. Guidelines of care for superficial mycotic infections of the skin: tinea corporis, tinea cruris, tinea faciei, tinea manuum, and tinea pedis. J Am Acad Dermatol 1996;34(2 pt 1):282–6.

[5] Taylor SC. Epidemiology of skin diseases in ethnic populations. Dermatol Clin 2003;21: 601–7.

[6] Adams BB. Tinea corporis gladiatorum. J Am Acad Dermatol 2002;47:286–90.

[7] Gupta AK, Chaudhry M, Elewski B. Tinea corporis, tinea cruris, tinea nigra, and piedra. Dermatol Clin 2003;21:395–400.

[8] Gupta AK, Cooper EA, Ryder JE, et al. Optimal management of fungal infections of the skin, hair, and nails. Am J Clin Dermatol 2004;5:225–37.

[9] Winokur RC, Dexter WW. Fungal infections and parasitic infections in sports. Phys Sports Med 2004;32:23–33.

[10] Budimulja U, Bramono K, Urip KS, et al. Once daily treatment with terbinafine 1% cream for one week is effective in the treatment of tinea corporis and cruris: a placebo controlled study. Mycoses 2001;44:300–6.

[11] Lester M. Ketoconazole 2 percent cream in the treatment of tinea pedis, tinea cruris, and tinea corporis. Cutis 1995;55:181–3.

[12] Faergemann J, Mork NJ, Haglund A, et al. A multicentre (double-blind) comparative study to assess the safety and efficacy of fluconazole and griseofulvin in the treatment of tinea corporis and tinea cruris. Br J Dermatol 1997;136:575–7.

[13] Pariser DM, Pariser RJ, Ruoff G, et al. Double-blind comparison of itraconazole and placebo in the treatment of tinea corporis and tinea cruris. J Am Acad Dermatol 1994;31:232–4.

[14] Farag A, Taha M, Halim S. One-week therapy with oral terbinafine in cases of tinea cruris/ corporis. Br J Dermatol 1994;131:684–6.

[15] Stary A, Sarnow E. Fluconazole in the treatment of tinea corporis and tinea cruris. Dermatology 1998;196:237–41.

[16] Crawfod F, Hart R, Bell-Syer S, et al. Topical treatments for fungal infections of the skin and nails of the foot. Cochrane Database Syst Rev 2000;2:CD001434.

[17] Bell-Syer SEM, Hart R, Crawford F, et al. Oral treatments for fungal infections of the skin of the foot. Cochrane Database Syst Rev 2002;2:CD003584.

[18] Kohl TD, Lisney M. Tinea gladiatorum: wrestling's emerging foe. Sports Med 2000;29: 439–47.

[19] Foster KW, Ghannoum MA, Elewski BE. Epidemiologic surveillance of cutaneous fungal infection in the United States from 1999 to 2002. J Am Acad Dermatol 2004;50: 748–52.

[20] Stiller MJ, Klein WP, Dorman RI, et al. Tinea corporis gladiatorum: an epidemic of *Trichophyton tonsurans* in student wrestlers. J Am Acad Dermatol 1992;27:632–3.

[21] Beller M, Gessner BD. An outbreak of tinea corporis gladiatorum on a high school wrestling team. J Am Acad Dermatol 1994;31:197–201.

[22] Hradil E, Hersle K, Nordin P, et al. An epidemic of tinea corporis caused by *Trychophyton tonsurans* among wrestlers in Sweden. Acta Derm Venereol (Stockh) 1995;75:305–6.

[23] Pique E, Copado R, Cabrera A, et al. An outbreak of tinea gladiatorum in Lanzarote. Clin Exp Dermatol 1999;24:7–9.

[24] Adams BB. Tinea corporis gladiatorum: a cross-sectional study. J Am Acad Dermatol 2000;43:1039–41.

[25] Kohl TD, Giesen DP, Moyer J Jr, et al. Tinea gladiatorum: Pennsylvania's experience. Clin J Sport Med 2002;12:165–71.

[26] Kohl TD, Martin DC, Berger MS. Comparison of topical and oral treatments for tinea gladiatorum. Clin J Sport Med 1999;9:161–6.

[27] Kohl TD, Martin DC, Nemeth R, et al. Fluconazole for the prevention and treatment of tinea gladiatorum. Pediatr Infect Dis J 2000;19:717–22.

[28] NCAA Rules Committee. "Appendix D: Skin Infections" in wrestling: 2006 rules and interpretations, 2005. Available at: http://www2.ncaa.org/media_and_events/ncaa_publications/playing_rules/. Accessed November 30, 2005.

[29] National Federation of State High School Associations, Sports Medicine Advisory Committee. Physician release for wrestler to participate with skin lesion. Available at: http://www.nfhs.org. Accessed March 15, 2006.

[30] Caputo R, De Boulle K, Del Rosso J, et al. Prevalence of superficial fungal infections among sports-active individuals: results from the Achilles survey, a review of the literature. J Eur Acad Dermatol Venereol 2001;15:312–6.

[31] Kamihama T, Kimura T, Hosokawa J-I, et al. Tinea pedis outbreak in swimming pools in Japan. Public Health 1997;111:249–53.

[32] Auger P, Marquis G, Joly J, et al. Epidemiology of tinea pedis in marathon runners: prevalence of occult athlete's foot. Mycoses 1993;36:35–41.

[33] Lacroix C, Baspeyras M, de La Salmoniere P, et al. Tinea pedis in European marathon runners. J Eur Acad Dermatol Venereol 2002;16:139–42.

[34] Strauss RH, Leizman DJ, Lanese RR, et al. Abrasive shirts may contribute to herpes gladiatorum among wrestlers. N Engl J Med 1989;320:598–9.

[35] Wheeler CE, Cabaniss WH. Epidemic cutaneous herpes simplex in wrestlers (herpes gladiatorum). JAMA 1965;194:145–9.

[36] Keilhofner M, McKinsey DS. Herpes gladiatorum in a high school wrestler. Mo Med 1988;85:723–5.

[37] Rosenbaum GS, Strampfer MJ, Cunha BA. Herpes gladiatorum in a male wrestler. Int J Dermatol 1990;29:141–2.

[38] US Department of Health and Human Services, Public Health Service. Herpes gladiatorum at a high school wrestling camp—Minnesota. MMWR Morb Mortal Wkly Rep 1990;39:69–71.

[39] Belongia EA, Goodman JL, Holland EJ, et al. An outbreak of herpes gladiatorum at a high school wrestling camp. N Engl J Med 1991;325:906–10.

[40] Holland EJ, Mahanti RL, Belongia EA, et al. Ocular involvement in an outbreak of herpes gladiatorum. Am J Ophthalmol 1992;114:680–4.

[41] Becker TM, Kodsi R, Bailey P, et al. Grappling with herpes: herpes gladiatorum. Am J Sports Med 1988;16:665–9.

[42] Anderson BJ. The epidemiology and clinical analysis of several outbreaks of herpes gladiatorum. Med Sci Sports Exerc 2003;11:1809–14.

[43] Barton SE, Ebel CW, Kirchner JT, et al. The clinical management of recurrent genital herpes: current issues and future prospects. Herpes 2002;9:15–20.

[44] Tyring SK, Douglas JM Jr, Corey L, et al. A randomized, placebo-controlled comparison of oral valacyclovir and acyclovir in immunocompetent patients with recurrent genital herpes infections. Arch Dermatol 1998;134:185–91.

[45] Anderson BJ. Valacyclovir to expedite the clearance of recurrent herpes gladiatorum. Clin J Sport Med 2005;15:364–6.

[46] Anderson BJ. The effectiveness of valacyclovir in preventing reactivation of herpes gladiatorum in wrestlers. Clin J Sport Med 1999;9:86–90.

[47] Niizeki K, Hashimoto K. Treatment of molluscum contagiosum with silver nitrate paste. Pediatr Dermatol 1999;16:395–7.

[48] Theos AU, Cummins R, Silverberg NB, et al. Effectiveness of imiquimod cream 5% for treating childhood molluscum contagiosum in a double-blind, randomized pilot trial. Cutis 2004;74:134–42.

[49] Syed TA, Goswami J, Ahmadpour OA, et al. Treatment of molluscum contagiosum in males with an analog of imiquimod 1% in cream: a placebo-controlled, double-blind study. J Dermatol 1998;25:309–13.

[50] Massing AM, Epstein WL. Natural history of warts. A two-year study. Arch Dermatol 1963;87:306–10.

[51] Gibbs S, Harvey I, Sterling J, et al. Local treatments for cutaneous warts: systematic review. BMJ 2002;325:461–7.

[52] Grussendorf-Conen EI, Jacobs S. Efficacy of imiquimod 5% cream in the treatment of recalcitrant warts in children. Pediatr Dermatol 2002;19:263–6.

[53] Grussendorf-Conen EI, Jacobs S, Rubben A, et al. Topical 5% imiquimod long-term treatment of cutaneous warts resistant to standard therapy modalities. Dermatology 2002;205: 139–45.

[54] Hengge UR, Esser S, Schultewolter T, et al. Self-administered topical 5% imiquimod for the treatment of common warts and molluscum contagiosum. Br J Dermatol 2000;143: 1026–31.

Clin Sports Med 26 (2007) 413–424

CLINICS IN SPORTS MEDICINE

ELSEVIER
SAUNDERS

HIV and the Athlete

Kelley L. Clem, MD, MS[a], James R. Borchers, MD[b],*

[a]Ohio Orthopedic Center of Excellence, 4605 Sawmill Road, Upper Arlington, OH 43220, USA
[b]The Ohio State University Sports Medicine Center, The Ohio State University, 2050 Kenny Road, Columbus, OH 43220, USA

Medical care of the athlete today continues to evolve, and athletes are participating in sport with a wide range of medical issues. In the last 30 years, perhaps the most important infectious disease issue facing the medical community is the emergence of HIV and AIDS. HIV/AIDS continues to be a worldwide health problem today, with millions of people around the world being affected. As the medical community has learned more about HIV/AIDS, treatment has improved and more people infected with HIV are living longer, productive lives. Athletes are not immune to the effects of HIV/AIDS, and there are many examples of athletes who have acquired the disease. Arthur Ashe was the first famous athlete to acknowledge infection with HIV and raised awareness about AIDS before he died from complications from the disease. Professional basketball player Earvin "Magic" Johnson had his career abbreviated by HIV/AIDS. He has, however, continued to participate in an active lifestyle while coping with the disease. As research has advanced the understanding of the natural history and treatment of HIV/AIDS, those dealing with the disease are living longer, leading sometimes-active lifestyles, and participating in sporting events. This understanding has raised awareness of competitive guidelines for those affected by HIV/AIDS. As a result, the sports medicine physician treating these individuals should have at least a basic understanding of the effects of exercise in the HIV/AIDS patient.

The first report of what was to become known as HIV/AIDS was published by the Centers for Disease Control and Prevention 25 years ago [1]. This report was a case series of *Pneumocystis carinii* pneumonia in five previously healthy young men in southern California. In addition to this atypical pneumonia, these men had low $CD4^+$ cell counts and similar constitutional complaints that helped to classify the disease known today as AIDS. Since this time, HIV/AIDS has become recognized as a worldwide pandemic, and the number of people affected by HIV/AIDS continues to rise not only in the United States

*Corresponding author. E-mail address: james.borchers@osumc.edu (J.R. Borchers).

0278-5919/07/$ – see front matter
doi:10.1016/j.csm.2007.04.012

but also around the world. It is estimated that in the United States, over 1 million persons are living with HIV/AIDS, with approximately 24% to 27% of affected individuals unaware of their infection [2]. This year (2006), an estimated 40,000 new cases are expected to occur in the United States alone [2]. As the number of infections rises, HIV/AIDS will continue to be an issue for athletes and those who care for them.

EPIDEMIOLOGY

HIV/AIDS continues to be a worldwide pandemic and has claimed the lives of more than 22 million persons, including more than 500,000 persons in the United States [1,2]. The number of new cases of AIDS has stabilized at approximately 40,000 cases annually in the United States since 1998 [2]. The rapid rise of diagnosed cases of HIV/AIDS in the United States in the 1980s peaked in 1992, and leveled off in 1998 [2]. From 1992 to 1998, secondary to early prevention and treatment advances, the number of HIV/AIDS cases decreased 47% across all demographic and transmission categories [2]. Most diagnosed HIV/AIDS cases occur in men, but an increasing proportion of cases are now being reported in women. Reported estimates from 2001 to 2004 suggest that 15% to 27% of diagnosed HIV/AIDS cases were in women and that the percentage is continuing an upward trend [1].

No ethnic group is spared from the effects of HIV/AIDS. From 1981 to 1995, the predominant ethnic group affected by HIV/AIDS was non-Hispanic whites (47%) [2]. Over time, however, racial and ethnic minorities have become disproportionately affected by the epidemic of HIV, with non-Hispanic African Americans (AA) accounting for 51% and Hispanics (H) accounting for 18% of the total cases reported from 2001 to 2004 [2]. The total case number of HIV/AIDS has decreased across all individuals at risk for HIV transmission; however, the case proportion of high-risk heterosexual contact has risen threefold, from 10% in 1991 to 1995 to 34% in 2001 to 2004 and is second only to male-to-male sexual contact (44%) [2]. The HIV/AIDS case rate for African Americans (76.3 per 100,000 population) and Hispanics (29.5 per 100,000 population) was 8.5 and 3.3 times higher, respectively, than the case rate for whites (9 per 100,000 population) [1]. From 2001 to 2004, African American men (131.6 per 100,000 population) had a case rate seven times that of white men (18.7 per 100,000 population) [1].

Survival rates among those living with HIV/AIDS have increased since 1996. The proportion of persons living 2 years after AIDS diagnosis has increased from 64% in 1981 to 1992 to 85% in 1996 to 2000 [1]. This increase is likely secondary to advances in drug treatment strategies and the development of effective prevention programs. There is a clear lack of epidemiologic information regarding athletes and HIV/AIDS. There is no study to date that has specifically investigated infection rates, risk, or transmission rates of HIV among competitive athletes. Therefore, it is unknown whether there is a difference among athletes compared with the general population regarding HIV/AIDS infection.

PATHOLOGY/PATHOPHYSIOLOGY

HIV is a retrovirus that (like all viruses) must use a host cell to replicate. HIV is in a subgroup of viruses called lentiviruses that are characterized by a latent period that may occur between initial infection and onset of disease [3]. Fig. 1 demonstrates the life cycle of HIV. Although not the direct cause of AIDS, the virus depletes $CD4^+$ T cells and, over time, waning immune function leads to increased incidence of opportunistic infections and ultimately the death of the affected individual. Infection of host cells involves proteins on the virus particle envelope (glycoprotein 120) that bind tightly to the CD4 protein of $CD4^+$ T cells [3]. When bound to the host cell, the virion injects viral RNA and a protein (reverse transcriptase) into the host cell cytoplasm using protein glycoprotein 40 [4]. The host cell is then programmed to replicate viral DNA.

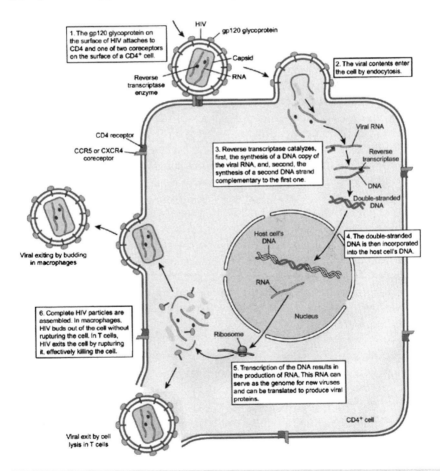

Fig. 1. Life cycle of the human immunodeficiency virus. gp, glycoprotein. (*From* Raven P, Johnson GB, Singer S, et al. Biology. 7th edition. New York: McGraw Hill, 2004; with permission of the Mcgraw-Hill Companies).

This viral DNA, which is compatible with human genetic material, is carried to the cell nucleus and spliced into the cell's native DNA by the HIV enzyme integrase. When incorporated into the cell's DNA, the virus becomes known as a provirus that may stay dormant for a long time. After the provirus is activated, the cell treats the HIV gene as its native genetic material coding for messenger RNA and manufactures HIV-related proteins and enzymes. These new proteins, enzymes, and genetic material gather together to form new viral particles that bud from the cell surface and are ready to infect other cells. In this fashion, the virus rapidly spreads through the body, disrupting the normal function of lymphocytes and T cell–mediated immunity. Although the main targets are T cells, macrophages and monocytes may also be affected. These cells are long lived and may act as a reservoir of HIV along with $CD4^+$ T cells [4].

As more cells become infected with HIV genetic material, T-cell immunity wanes and opportunistic infections may occur. Although these opportunistic infections may be seen at any level of CD4 cell count, the incidence of serious and life-threatening infection increases dramatically at $CD4^+$ counts less than 200/mL [5]. CD4 thresholds of 200/mL, 100/mL, and 50/mL have been established to demarcate risk of *Pneumocystis jiroveci*, *Toxoplasma gondii*, and *Mycobacterium avium* complex, respectively, and are indications for prophylaxis [5,6]. Consensus guidelines recommend obtaining plasma HIV-1 RNA levels in addition to $CD4^+$ cell counts when considering therapy because mortality data have indicated that patients who have HIV-1 RNA levels greater than 100,000 copies per milliliter are at increased risk of disease progression independent of CD4 cell count [5,6]. Near-uniform findings that disease progression and mortality are worse when therapy is delayed until CD4 cell counts are less than 200/mL support the recommendation to initiate treatment at counts higher than this number. Patients who present with initial CD4 cell counts less than 200/mL should be offered therapy as soon as a baseline evaluation is completed. Persons who have CD4 cell counts above 350/mL generally may be observed because data indicate similar results with and without therapy. As previously described, however, those who have plasma HIV-1 RNA counts above 100,000/mL are at increased risk of disease progression and should be offered therapy [5].

DIAGNOSIS

Although an affected individual may have been HIV positive for some time, he or she may not recognize the symptoms of the disease. Common nonspecific signs and symptoms may be the first presentation of HIV infection. Lethargy, lack of energy, repeated or prolonged illness, and high-risk behaviors are symptoms and signs that should prompt inclusion of HIV in the differential diagnosis. An athlete may have mild symptoms and otherwise present with a complaint of recent poor performances. Obtaining a detailed history from an athlete may help differentiate a less serious illness from a more serious disease such as HIV/AIDS. Otherwise, a thorough history and physical should prompt a workup that includes testing for HIV. When testing returns a positive result, proper referral can be made to an HIV specialist for further testing, counseling, and treatment of the athlete. Some high-risk sports may require pre-participation screening for HIV. For example, the state of Nevada currently mandates testing for HIV during prefight physicals. Although only a few individuals have tested positive before a competition, the fact that the Nevada Boxing Commission has acknowledged the potential dangers of HIV infection in an athlete illustrates the concern for HIV transmission risk in boxing.

HIV transmission risk is considered rare in athletic competition. Transmission of HIV occurs through sexual contact, contact with blood and blood products, contamination of a wound with infected blood, or contact with mucous membranes [5]. There is no evidence of HIV transmission through casual contact, including contact during athletic competition. The virus may be present in a variety of body fluids, but blood poses the most risk during athletic activities. Tears, sweat, urine, sputum, vomitus, saliva, and respiratory droplets have not been implicated in transmission of HIV. Although the risk of HIV transmission is unlikely in athletic competition, the possibility of it occurring should be considered in high-risk sports.

TREATMENT

Advances in HIV/AIDS treatment have decreased the morbidity and mortality associated with the disease. In patients whose CD4 cell counts are between 200/mL and 350/mL, the recommendation to start therapy should be made on an individual basis. One study has suggested that 275/mL is a level at which HIV is likely to progress and may be a threshold to initiate therapy [5,7].

Therapy regimens involve multiple antiretroviral medications, with the goal to suppress plasma HIV-1 titers to less than 50 copies per milliliter [8]. There are five drug classes represented by 21 drugs and five fixed-combination therapies currently approved and available in the United States for treatment of HIV [5].

Two non-nucleoside reverse transcriptatse inhibitors–efavirenz or nevirapine–used in combination with two nucleoside analog reverse transcriptase inhibitors or one nucleoside analog and one nucleotide analog reverse transcriptase inhibitor, are frequently used. The combination of efavirenz and the nucleotide-nucleoside component tenofovir-emtricitabine has been found more effective in suppressing plasma HIV-1 RNA and increasing CD4 cell counts than the combination of efavirenz and zidovudine-lamivudine [9]. Alternative combination therapies are available that involve protease inhibitors; however, side effects of these drugs make them less attractive for primary use. Metabolic derangements such as metabolic syndrome have been linked to protease inhibitors, and nucleoside analogs have been linked to lipoatrophy and mitochondrial toxicity. Increased cardiovascular risk, especially myocardial infarction, has been associated with antiretroviral therapy [10]. These side effects, along with central nervous system, gastrointestinal, and integumentary system effects, may also increase symptoms of fatigue, depressive moods, and anxiety seen in patients who have HIV/AIDS.

It is unknown whether athletes experience these side effects with the same incidence as the general population or whether the effects are as severe. Certainly, high-level athletic performance could be adversely affected; however, exercise has been used to lessen the severity of symptoms in other chronic disease processes, and the benefits of a regular training program may offset the potential side effects of treatment.

EXERCISE TRAINING AND HIV

As the number of individuals diagnosed with HIV continues to grow, it is likely that these individuals will want to participate in healthy lifestyles, including participating in athletic endeavors. Positive physical and psychologic benefits of exercise have been demonstrated for individuals who have other medical diagnoses [11–18].

The effects of exercise have been used to treat symptoms of fatigue, depression, nausea, and anxiety in patients who have chronic disease such as fibromyalgia, cancer, chronic fatigue syndrome, Hodgkin's disease, and cardiovascular disease, with positive results [11]. The dose of exercise has varied but, in general, prolonged training programs have consisted of 8 to 12 weeks of aerobic activity, 3 to 5 days/week, at 60% to 85% maximal heart rate. Even single bouts of exercise have been demonstrated to reduce fatigue and increase vigor in healthy individuals [11,12]. Numerous studies have shown exercise benefits with regard to anxiety and depression in patients suffering from chronic disease. These include patients who have cardiovascular disease, chronic obstructive pulmonary disease, multiple sclerosis, diabetes, and fibromyalgia. Reductions of anxiety in breast cancer patients have been seen after only 15 minutes of moderate-intensity cycling [13]. Exercise programs have demonstrated similar effects of elevating positive mood states, energy, and general well-being not only in healthy individuals but also in cancer populations [14,15]. Exercise programs have also been suggested for potential analgesic-like effects. Improvements of pain tolerance and tender-point pain pressure threshold have been demonstrated after exercise training programs [11,14,19].

The data supporting that exercise has a beneficial effect on negative physical states and a positive effect on positive and negative psychologic states are clear. Prolonged exercise programs have demonstrated the benefits of reducing fatigue, nausea, pain perception, dyspnea, depression, and anxiety and of increasing mood, vigor, and well-being across multiple populations. As research continues in this area, it is hoped that patients who have HIV/AIDS will respond similarly. Emerging literature suggests that short bouts of exercise and prolonged training have no adverse physiologic effects in patients who have HIV/AIDS.

Exercise interventions performed in the early 1990s by LaPierre and colleagues [21] reported increased CD4$^+$ cell counts with aerobic exercise training. These data have not been reproduced. Subsequent studies by Smith and colleagues [22], Rigsby and colleagues [23], and Roubenoff and Wilson [24] that looked at resistance training or aerobic training did not demonstrate an adverse effect on $CD4^+$ cell counts or viral load. MacArthur and colleagues [25] in 1993 associated lower $CD4^+$ cell counts with exercise noncompliance. Perna and colleagues [26] in 1999 demonstrated similar results. The data reported by LaPierre [20] were from a lower socioeconomic class and it was suggested that exercise may have played a role in stress reduction, thus the rise in $CD4^+$ cells reflected a normalizing of stress-induced $CD4^+$ cell depletion [21]. For HIV-infected individuals who wish to pursue a physically active lifestyle and perhaps participate in competitive athletics, no adverse effects to $CD4^+$ cell counts are evident.

Early studies concerned with the wasting effects of HIV/AIDS focused on the ability of patients who have HIV/AIDS to complete aerobic and resistance training programs and to determine physiologic responses. Results were consistently positive. Increases in aerobic capacity (maximum oxygen consumption [$\dot{V}o_2max$]) and lactate threshold were seen after aerobic endurance exercise training programs [11,26,27]. Increases in lean body mass, strength, and physical function have been consistently demonstrated with resistance training programs in HIV-positive patients [11,16–18,28]. There is not yet clear evidence that resistance training can reduce the effects of antiretroviral therapy–associated lipodystrophy; however, there is ample evidence that resistance training is not harmful and that participation in a resistance training program is beneficial for the HIV-infected individual.

Extensive literature exists to support the fact that HIV-infected individuals may respond to physical training in a similar manner to healthy individuals. In HIV-infected individuals, there have not been adverse effects such as decreased $CD4^+$ cell counts or increased plasma HIV RNA levels. Thus, it has been generally assumed that participation in moderate-intensity training programs is not detrimental to these individuals.

Acute bouts of high-intensity exercise in healthy individuals have been shown to activate the immune system, leading to leukocytosis, neutrophilia, lymphopenia, and increased respiratory viral infections. Production of the inflammatory cytokines interleukin 1β and tumor necrosis factor α is increased, which may increase HIV replication. Roubenoff and colleagues [28] in 1999 investigated the effect of a single bout of acute exercise on plasma HIV RNA levels in 25 patients who had HIV infection. Absolute neutrophil counts, serum creatine phosphokinase, and urinary 3-methylhistidine were increased in response to exercise, indicating a mild acute-phase response [28]. Mean plasma HIV RNA levels were elevated at baseline in 22 of 25 subjects and did not show further increase after exercise [28]. In 3 subjects who had undetectable plasma HIV RNA levels, small but nonsignificant increases were seen [28]. It was concluded that acute bouts of exercise at moderate to high intensity is not associated with an increase of HIV viral load [28]. Because regular exercise has not been shown to activate the acute-phase response and the fact that there is no elevation in viral loads with acute bouts of exercise suggest that exercise training is safe in HIV-infected individuals. Stringer and colleagues [27] demonstrated similar results in

1998. Thirty-four subjects who had HIV infection were randomized into three groups: one control and two exercise groups. The exercise groups were (1) moderate intensity, 80% of lactate threshold work rate; and (2) high intensity, 50% of difference between lactate threshold and $\dot{V}O_2$max. The subjects trained three times per week for 6 weeks. The total work performed was the same for both groups. After the training period, immune indices and plasma HIV RNA were unchanged. $CD4^+$ cell counts tended to increase with moderate-to-heavy exercise, but these were nonsignificant changes. A *Candida* skin test in the moderate-intensity group demonstrated a significantly more robust response. Thus, there was no indication of worsening immune function with high-intensity exercise and, as demonstrated in previous studies, there were improvements in aerobic function as measured by $\dot{V}O_2$max.

The above studies suggest that participation in exercise—acute or regular and moderate or high intensity—is safe for those infected with HIV. Exercise programs not only improve physiologic function but have also been demonstrated to improve quality of life. There have been numerous athletes diagnosed with HIV, and the literature to date suggests that although it is safe to continue to exercise, participation in competitive events may present a hazard to other participants. Table 1 is a limited summary of the literature regarding exercise and exercise-related benefits in a variety of patients, including those affected with HIV.

SAFETY OF PARTICIPATION

The issue of safe participation has been addressed by multiple leading sports medicine organizations. The American Medical Society for Sports Medicine and the American Orthopaedic Society for Sports Medicine issued a joint position statement regarding blood-borne diseases and athletic competition that addresses epidemiology, transmission, education, and preventive measures for blood-borne pathogens [29]. Although there are no epidemiologic studies assessing transmission of HIV during athletic activity, the risk of HIV transmission in the National Football League has been conservatively estimated at less than 1 in 1 million games [29]. In sports in which significant blood exposures to open wounds could take place, however, the theoretic chance for HIV transmission is not zero.

Preventive education is paramount in preventing the spread of blood-borne pathogens. Sports medicine practitioners, athletic trainers, coaches, and officials play important roles in educational activities. Regarding HIV, athletes should be educated in a clear manner of the risk of HIV transmission through sexual contact and high-risk behaviors including alcohol and drug abuse that may lead to increased risk of exposure. Athletes should also be advised not to share personal items that may be contaminated with blood, such as razors, toothbrushes, and nail clippers.

During competition, athletes should be made aware that it is in their best interest to report injuries in a timely manner and to seek first aid for bleeding injuries. This is a common sense approach; however, it may need to be repeated to ensure compliance.

Table 1
Studies of exercise and related effects

Author [Reference]	Research question	Outcome	Level of evidence
Ciccolo et al 2004 [11]	Systematic review of exercise and chronic illnesses including HIV	Exercise training may improve quality of life	2a
Morgan, 1985 [12]	Systematic review of psychogenic factors affecting exercise	Psychogenic factors can significantly influence exercise metabolism	2a
Bartholomew & Miller, 2002 [14]	Mastery hypothesis for affective benefits of acute exercise	High-performance participants reported greater and longer effects of exercise throughout recovery	1b
Burnham & Wilcox, 2002 [15]	Effect of aerobic exercise on physiologic and psychologic function in patients rehabilitating from cancer treatment	Statistically significant increases in aerobic capacity and lower-body flexibility, a significant decrease in body fat, a significant increase in quality of life, and a measure of energy in the exercise group compared with the control group	1b
Bopp et al 2004 [21]	Association of physical activity and CD4$^+$ cell count and viral load	Inverse relationship of activity and viral load, no relationship with cell counts	3b
Roubenoff et al 1999 [28]	Effect of single, high-intensity exercise on plasma HIV RNA levels	No significant increase of plasma HIV RNA levels with exercise	3b
Stringer et al 1998 [27]	Aerobic training effect on fitness, immune indices, and quality of life	Improved aerobic function and quality-of-life markers No change of immune indices	2b

To minimize the risk of blood-borne pathogen transmission during athletic events, the American Medical Society for Sports Medicine and the American Orthopaedic Society for Sports Medicine recommend the following practices:

1. Existing wounds and skin rashes should be properly prepared.
2. Equipment and supplies should be available for compliance with universal precautions.
3. Those who have uncontrolled bleeding or an uncovered wound should be recognized and removed from competition. Blood-saturated clothing should be removed.

4. The athlete is responsible for wearing protective equipment.
5. Minor cuts and abrasions should be cleaned and dressed.
6. Care providers should follow universal precautions.
7. Personal airway devices should be made available to care providers.
8. Equipment contaminated with blood should be cleaned immediately with disinfecting solution.
9. Wounds should be re-evaluated post competition.
10. HBV immunization should be considered for health care team members.

Most universities have in place policies and procedures regarding blood-borne pathogens including HIV.

When caring for athletes infected with HIV, it is important that they have access to knowledgeable HIV-related medical care, counseling services dealing with the psychologic aspects of the disease, and maintenance of confidentiality as dictated by medical ethics and legal statues. The decision to participate in competitive athletics should be made on an individual basis. This decision should take into account the individual's current state of health and physical fitness, the nature and intensity of the sport, the potential contribution of stress from competition, and the potential risk for HIV transmission.

Currently, HIV infection alone is insufficient grounds to prohibit athletic participation in competition. There have been challenges in the judicial system that have contested a school's decision to prohibit an HIV-positive individual from competing in athletics. Most are successful. When there is a likelihood of blood exposure to an open wound, however, the courts have upheld the school's decision to restrict participation [30].

SUMMARY

Advances in medical care and therapeutics have resulted in longer symptom-free survival and higher quality of life of those affected with HIV. With high-profile athletes being infected with HIV and drawing attention to HIV/AIDS, this in turn may lead to increased participation of HIV-infected individuals in competitive athletics. Society and the medical community will need to address several issues: (1) Is it safe for those who have very low or negligible viral counts to participate in sports with possible body-fluid exposures? (2) At what level is it safe to allow participation? (3) As HIV/AIDS progresses to a chronic disease that requires monitoring, can physicians safely recommend that an affected athlete participate at high levels of athletic activity without risk to the athlete or to other participants?

Continuing research on the effects of exercise on long-term survival and viral pathophysiology are important, especially as treatments become more effective in driving down viral counts, some to near-unmeasurable levels. To date, there is a paucity of epidemiologic studies regarding HIV and transmissibility in athletic competition. With the number of asymptomatic HIV-infected individuals likely to increase, the investigation of exercise and HIV disease transmission will be an important area of study in the near future.

References

[1] Twenty-five years of HIV/AIDS—United States, 1981–2005. MMWR Morb Mortal Wkly Rev 2006;55(21):589–92.

[2] Epidemiology of HIV/AIDS—United States, 1981–2005. MMWR Morb Mortal Wkly Rev 2006;55(21):589–92.

[3] Greene WC, Peterlin BM. Molecular insights into HIV biology. HIV InSite Knowledge Base Chapter; February 2003.

[4] Hare CB. Clinical overview of HIV disease. HIV InSite Knowledge Base Chapter; January 2006.

[5] Hammer SM. Management of newly diagnosed HIV infection. N Engl J Med 2005;353: 1702–10.

[6] Egger M, May M, Chene G, et al. Prognosis of HIV-1 infected patients starting highly active antiretroviral therapy: a collaborative analysis of prospective studies. Lancet 2002;360: 119–29.

[7] Ahdieh-Grant L, Yamashita TE, Phair JP, et al. When to initiate highly active antiretroviral therapy: a cohort approach. Am J Epidemiol 2003;157:738–46.

[8] Bartlett JA, Fath MJ, DeMasi R, et al. An updated meta-analysis of triple combination therapy in antiretroviral-naïve HIV-infected adults. Presented at the 12th Conference on Retroviruses and Opportunistic Infections. Boston, February 22–25, 2005.

[9] Pozniak AL, Gallant JE, DeJesus E, et al. Superior outcome for tenofovir DF, emtricitabine and efavirenz compared to fixed dose zidovudine/lamivudine and efavirenz in antiretroviral-naïve patients. Presented at the 3rd IAS Conference on Pathogenesis and Treatment. Rio de Janeiro, July 24–27, 2005.

[10] Friis-Moller N, Sabin CA, Weber R, et al. Combination antiretroviral therapy and the risk of myocardial infarction. N Engl J Med 2003;349:1993–2003.

[11] Ciccolo JT, Jowers EM, Bartholomew JB. The benefits of exercise for quality of life in the post-HAART era. Sports Med 2004;34(8):487–99.

[12] Morgan WP. Affective benefence of vigorous physical activity. Med Sci Exerc 1985;177: 94–100.

[13] Mock V, Dow KH, Meares CJ, et al. Effects of exercise on fatigue, physical functioning, and emotional distress during radiation therapy for breast cancer. Oncol Nurs Forum 1997;24: 991–1000.

[14] Bartholomew JB, Miller BM. Affective responses to an aerobic dance class: the impact of perceived performance. Res Q Exerc Sport 2002;73:301–9.

[15] Burnham TR, Wilcox A. Effects of exercise on physiological and psychological variables in cancer survivors. Med Sci Sports Exerc 2002;34:1863–7.

[16] Roubenoff R, McDermott A, Weiss L, et al. Short-term progressive resistance training increases strength and lean body mass in adults infected with human immunodeficiency virus. AIDS 1999;13:231–9.

[17] Agin D, Kotler DP, Papandreou D, et al. Effects of whey protein and resistance exercise on body composition and muscle strength I women with HIV infection. Ann N Y Acad Sci 2000;904:607–9.

[18] Agin D, Gallagher D, Wang J, et al. Effects of whey protein and resistance exercise on body cell mass, muscle strength and quality of life in women with HIV. AIDS 2001;15:2431–40.

[19] Busch A, Schachter CL, Pelosi PM, et al. Exercise for treating fibromyalgia syndrome. Cochrane Database Syst Rev 2002;3:CD003786.

[20] LaPierre AR, Antoni MH, Schneiderman N, et al. Exercise intervention attenuates the emotional distress and natural killer cell decrements following notification of positive serologic status for HIV-1. Biofeedback Self Regul 1990;15:229–42.

[21] Bopp CM, Phillips KD, Fulk LJ, et al. Physical activity and immunity in HIV-infected individuals. AIDS Care 2004;16(3):387–93.

[22] Smith BA, Neidig JL, Nickel JT, et al. Aerobic exercise; effects on parameters related to fatigue, dyspnea, weight, body composition in HIV-infected adults. AIDS 2001;15:693–701.

[23] Rigsby LW, Dichman RK, Jackson AW, et al. Effects of exercise training on men seropositive for the human immunodeficiency virus-1. Med Sci Sports Exerc 1992;24:6–12.

[24] Roubenoff R, Wilson IB. Effect of resistance training on self reported physical functioning in HIV infection. Med Sci Exerc 2001;33:1811–7.

[25] MacArthur RD, Levine SD, Birk TJ. Supervised exercise training improves cardiopulmonary fitness in HIV-infected persons. Med Sci Sports Exerc 1993;25:684–8.

[26] Perna F, LaPerriere A, Klimas N, et al. Cardiopulmonary and CD4 cell changes in response to exercise training in early symptomatic HIV infection. Med Sci Sports Exerc 1999;31: 973–9.

[27] Stringer WW, Berezovskaya M, O'Brien WA, et al. The effect of exercise training on aerobic fitness, immune indices, and quality of life in HIV+ patients. Med Sci Sports Exerc 1998;30(1):11–6.

[28] Roubenoff R, Skolnik PR, Shevitz A, et al. Effect of single bout of acute exercise on plasma human immunodeficiency virus RNA levels. J Appl Physiol 1999;86(4):1197–201.

[29] American Medical Society for Sports Medicine and American Orthopedic Society of Sports Medicine Position Statement. Human immunodeficiency virus (HIV) and other blood-borne pathogens in sports. Available at: www.newamssm.org/hiv.html. Accessed January 2006.

[30] HIV-positive boy can be barred from group karate lessons. AIDS Policy Law 1999;14(4): 1–8.

Clin Sports Med 26 (2007) 425–431

CLINICS IN SPORTS MEDICINE

ELSEVIER
SAUNDERS

Blood-Borne Infections

Jason J. Pirozzolo, DO[a], Donald C. LeMay, DO[b],*

[a]CentraCare Hospital, 60001 Vineland Avenue, Suite 108, Orlando, FL 32819, USA
[b]The Ohio State University, Division of Sports Medicine, OSU Sports Medicine Center,
Martha Moorehouse Building, 3rd Floor, 2050 Kenny Road, Columbus, OH 43221, USA

Blood-borne infections continue to be a major problem throughout the world. Hepatitis B virus (HBV), hepatitis C virus (HCV), and HIV are the most common pathogens encountered. Although human T-lymphotropic virus 1, hepatitis G virus, cytomegalovirus, Creutzfeldt-Jakob disease, leshmaniasis, malaria, Chagas' disease, babesiosis, and toxoplasmosis are all infections that may be transmitted by similar routes, this article focuses on HBV and HCV as being the most prevalent in athletics.

According to the World Health Organization, over 350 million people worldwide are chronically infected with HBV. The Centers for Disease Control and Prevention (CDC) has documented that 1.25 million people in the United States are infected with HBV [1]. In 2000, approximately 521,000 deaths were attributed to HBV-related illnesses. It is also estimated that 180 million people worldwide are infected with HCV, with 130 million being chronic carriers. In the United States, 1.8% of the population is affected with HCV, with 3.8 million exposed and 2.7 million chronically affected. HCV and HBV are major causes of acute hepatitis and chronic liver disease, including primary hepatocellular carcinoma and cirrhosis, which eventually leads to liver failure [2].

MECHANISM OF TRANSMISSION

Blood-borne infections are transmitted in athletes by similar mechanisms as in the general population, including direct blood contact from one individual to another from injured skin or a mucous membrane. There is a low risk of transmission during sporting activities from bleeding wounds or exudative skin injury of an infected athlete to the injured skin or mucous membrane of another athlete. Obviously, the risk may be higher with contact and collision sports such as wrestling and boxing. Athletes participating in activities that require very little physical contact such as gymnastics, cheerleading, baseball, and tennis are at a substantially lower risk [3].

*Corresponding author. E-mail address: donald.lemay@osumc.edu (D.C. LeMay).

0278-5919/07/$ – see front matter
doi:10.1016/j.csm.2007.04.010

As with the general population, blood-borne infections can also be transmitted through blood doping and drug abuse. In 1993, Yesalis and colleagues [4] reported that approximately 1 million people were currently using or had a history of using anabolic androgenic steroids. Approximately 50% used the drug intramuscularly, and 25% admitted to sharing needles. An athlete who shares a needle is at increased risk of contracting blood-borne viruses. HIV infection was reported in three Austrian bodybuilders; each of these documented cases was a result of sharing needles to inject anabolic androgenic steroids [5–8].

Blood-borne infections have also shown to be transmitted through sexual contact. The highest risk for transmission is homosexual sex with men and heterosexual sex with multiple partners. Heterosexual contact with an infected individual continues to be the most common method of HBV transmission [9]. There is widespread speculation that male athletes participate in riskier sexual activities, have more partners, and have a greater prevalence of sexually transmitted diseases, but there is no definitive evidence to support this [10,11].

Finally, one must take into consideration the traveling athlete. Risk factors for HBV infection include travel to regions with endemic hepatitis, which is important when risk stratifying athletes [9].

HEPATITIS B VIRUS

HBV is a double-stranded circular DNA virus in the Hepadnaviridae family. The DNA is enclosed in a nucleocapsid (core antigen) and surrounded by a spherical envelope (surface antigen). These antigens, in addition to their corresponding antibodies, are useful in determining past, current, or chronic HBV infections (Box 1).

Box 1: Laboratory markers for HBV

Hepatitis B surface antigen (HBsAg): present in acute or chronic infection

Hepatitis B surface antibody (anti-HBs): marker of immunity acquired through natural HBV infection, vaccination, or passive antibody (immune globulin)

Hepatitis B core antibody (anti-HBc):

  IgM—indicative of infection in the previous six months

  IgG—indicative of more distant HBV infection that may have been cleared by the immune system or that may persist; positive HBsAg and anti-HBc

  IgG—indicative of persistent chronic HBV infection

Hepatitis B e antigen (HBeAg): correlates with a high level of viral replication; often called a "marker of infectivity"

Hepatitis B e antibody (anti-HBe): correlates with low rates of viral replication

HBV DNA: correlates with active replication; useful in monitoring response to treatment of HBV infection, especially in HBeAg-negative mutants

From Lin KW, Kirchner JT, Hepatitis B. American Family Physician 2004;69:76; with permission.

In the athletic setting, there have been numerous documented HBV outbreaks. In 1982, a case report was presented that recognized 5 of 10 members of a Japanese high school sumo wrestling club who contracted hepatitis B during a single year. It was suggested that these cases were spread through skin cuts and abrasions during wrestling. These individuals continued to wrestle despite active bleeding from their skin wounds [12]. In 2000, an outbreak of HBV in an American football team was reported in which 11 of 65 athletes over a 19-month period were found to have HBV. Again, contact with the open wounds of an HBV carrier was thought to be the precipitating factor [13].

The risk of transmission of HBV is approximately 50 to 100 times higher than the risk of transmission of HIV. HBV is also more stable when exposed to the environment. HBV is resistant to alcohol, some detergents, and has been shown to flourish on environmental surfaces for over 7 days [14]. The estimated risk of transmission of HBV after a percutaneous exposure in health care workers is calculated to be 2% to 40%. This risk compares to 0.2% to 0.5% risk of transmission for HIV. The theoretic risk of transmission of HBV in sport has been calculated based on the estimated prevalence of HBV among athletes. These data reveal a risk that is between one transmission in every 10,000 to 50,000 games to one transmission in every 850,000 to 4.25 million games [15–17]. Another study described the prevalence of HBV infection in athletes as being no different from blood donors of the same age [18,19].

Although HBV infection may present subclinically in up to 70% of adults, many individuals present with nausea, anorexia, low-grade fever, or abdominal pain. Other systemic symptoms may include myalgia, urticaria, and joint pain. These symptoms may last anywhere from 1 to 3 months [11].

Chronic HBV is diagnosed following 6 months of a positive hepatitis B surface antigen. Approximately 12% of patients who have chronic HBV infection go on to develop liver cirrhosis or hepatocellular carcinoma each year [20]. Patients considered for treatment of chronic HBV are typically started on immune modulators such as recombinant interferon alfa-2b or antivirals that directly inhibit HBV replication, including lamivudine and adefovir dipivoxil [21].

HEPATITIS C VIRUS

The HCV genome is a single-stranded, positive-sense RNA molecule. Following an average incubation period of 6 to 7 weeks, almost 70% of patients who have acute HCV infection have no discernible symptoms, 20% to 30% present with jaundice, and 10% to 20% have nonspecific symptoms such as loss of appetite, fatigue, and abdominal pain [22–24].

The risk of HCV infection is substantial in intravenous drug users. Alter and colleagues reported that approximately 50% to 80% of users were anti-HCV positive within 12 months of initial use [25]. HCV transmission has been reported in multiple injectors of anabolic androgenic steroids. In 1994, Morrison and colleagues [26–28] observed one case of exposure to HCV among five steroid injectors. Another report described three soccer players from a single amateur club who were infected with HCV as a direct result of sharing a syringe to inject intravenous vitamin complexes [5].

The incidence of anti-HCV seroconversion among health care workers after accidental needle stick or sharp surgical instruments exposures was 1.8%. The risk of transmitting HCV through sexual activity is currently being debated. Lifetime risk for sexual transmission of HCV in monogamous couples appears to be less than 1%. The general data suggest that if it does occur, it does so at a very low frequency. When transmission occurs, however, up to 85% of patients eventually develop chronic HCV [25].

> Diagnosing the HCV infection is accomplished by obtaining a serum anti-HCV antibody (at least 99% sensitive and specific) or HCV RNA. Routine screening is recommended by the CDC for individuals who have the following risk factors:
> 1. History of intravenous drug use
> 2. Blood transfusion or organ transplant before 1989
> 3. Recipient of clotting factors before 1987
> 4. Long-term hemodialysis

Routine screening of asymptomatic patients should include enzyme immunoassay or anti-HCV and confirmatory testing if needed [29]. Patients who have chronic HCV tend to present with persistently elevated alanine aminotransferase levels, detectable HCV RNA, and portal fibrosis. Interferon treatment is generally recommended for these patients to delay the progression to cirrhosis [30–33].

PREVENTION

Today, with the increase of infected athletes in competitive situations, prevention has become an integral part of athletic health care. As indicated earlier, the primary method of transmission of blood-borne infections in athletes is not through sports activity but by the same mechanisms as in the general population. Therefore, much of the effort to prevent these infections among athletes has been to educate all involved participants.

"Universal precautions" dealing with blood and body fluids have been developed to minimize the risk of blood-borne pathogen transmission during athletic events. In 1999, the American Academy of Pediatrics published an extensive series of recommendations titled, "Human Immunodeficiency Virus and Other Blood-Borne Viral Pathogens in the Athletic Setting" [28]. This guideline has been used as the bases for multiple organizations, including the National Collegiate Athletic Association, to formulate recommendations to curve the spread of blood-borne infections in the athletic population. These guidelines include caring for the student athlete and cleansing and disinfecting environmental surfaces. Caring for the athlete includes the following recommendations:

- The physician should respect the right of infected athletes to confidentiality.
- Athletes should not be tested for blood-borne pathogens because they are sports participants.

- Physicians are encouraged to counsel athletes who are infected with HIV, HBV, or HCV that they have a very small risk of infecting other competitors. Infected athletes should consider choosing a sport in which this risk is apparently relatively low.
- Clinicians and the staff of athletic programs should aggressively promote HBV immunization among athletes and among coaches, athletic trainers, equipment handlers, laundry personnel, and any other persons at risk of exposure to athletes' blood as an occupational hazard. All athletes should receive HBV vaccinations.
- Each coach and athletic trainer must receive training in first aid and emergency care and in the prevention of transmission of blood-borne pathogens in the athletic setting.
- Coaches and members of the health care team should educate athletes about the risks of transmission of HIV and other blood-borne pathogens through sexual activity and needle sharing during the use of illicit drugs, including anabolic steroids.
- Athletes should practice good personal hygiene and be educated not to share personal items such as razors, toothbrushes, and nail clippers that might be contaminated with blood.
- In some states, depending on state law, schools may need to comply with Occupational Safety and Health Administration (OSHA) regulations for the prevention of transmission of blood-borne pathogens. The athletic program must determine what rules apply. Compliance with OSHA regulations is a reasonable and recommended precaution even if this is not specifically required by the state.

The caring of athletes, environmental surfaces, and equipment should be done by personnel who are properly trained in first aid and standard precautions. Personal protective equipment, antiseptics, antimicrobial wipes, bandages, medical equipment, and properly labeled waste receptacles should be

---

Box 2: Preventative precautions with body fluids

To avoid contact with blood or body fluids, latex gloves should be used.

Exposed wounds or damaged skin of athletes and caregivers should be covered.

Athletes who have active bleeding should be taken out of competition immediately. The wound area should be cleansed and covered with an occlusive dressing before returning to competition.

Athletes should report any injury immediately.

If rescue breathing is needed at an athletic venue, proper equipment such as an CPR bag valve mask should be used. If proper equipment is not available, then mouth-to-mouth rescue breathing is appropriate.

Spray contaminated surfaces with chemical germicides or freshly prepared bleach solutions (diluted 1:10 bleach/water).

Proper techniques should be used when dealing with contaminated equipment and laundry, whether or not it has noticeable blood or body fluids.

available at all training rooms and sporting events as needed to deal with body fluids and bleeding athletes. In addition, learning how and when wounds should be cleaned and covered and when to return an athlete to competition is paramount (Box 2).

SUMMARY

Athletes are a high-risk population due to travel, the environment, and lifestyle behaviors. Knowledge and awareness of appropriate preventative strategies are essential for all student-athletes. The emphasis of blood-borne pathogen prevention for the student-athlete and the health care team should be on traditional transmission routes and off-the-field behavior of athletes because experts believe that field transmission of blood-borne pathogens is minimal.

References

[1] Available at: http://www.cdc.gov/ncidod/diseases/hepatitis/b/fact.htm.
[2] Available at: http://www.who.int/immunization/topics/hepatitis_c/en/index.html.
[3] Kordi R, Wallace WA. Blood borne infections in sport: risks of transmission, methods of prevention, and recommendations for hepatitis B vaccination. Br J Sports Med 2004;38: 678–84.
[4] Yesalis CE, Kennedy NJ, Kopstein AN, et al. Anabolic-androgenic steroid use in the United States. JAMA 1993;8:1217–21.
[5] Parana R, Lyra L, Trepo C. Intravenous vitamin complexes used in sporting activities and transmission of HCV in Brazil. Am J Gastroenterol 1999;94:857–8.
[6] Henrion R, Mandelbrot L, Delfieu D. HIV contamination after injections of anabolic steroids. Presse Med 1992;8:218.
[7] Sklarek HM, Mantovani RP, Erens E, et al. AIDS in a bodybuilder using anabolic steroids. N Engl J Med 1984;311:1701.
[8] Scott MJ, Scott MJJ. HIV infection associated with injections of anabolic steroids. JAMA 1989;14:207–8.
[9] Available at: http://www.who.int/mediacentre/factsheets/fs204/en/.
[10] Trost SG, Levin S, Pate RR. Sport, physical activity and other health behaviours in children and adolescents. In: Armstrong N, Van Mechelen W, editors. Paediatric exercise science and medicine. Oxford (UK): Oxford University Press; 2000. p. 295–310.
[11] Lee WM. Hepatitis B virus infection. N Engl J Med 1997;337:1733–45.
[12] Kashiwagi S, Hayashi J, Ikematsu H, et al. An outbreak of hepatitis B in members of a high school sumo wrestling club. JAMA 1982;248:213–4.
[13] Tobe K, Matsuura K, Ogura T, et al. Horizontal transmission of hepatitis B virus among players of an American football team. Arch Intern Med 2000;160:2541–5.
[14] Beltrami EM, Williams IT, Shapiro CN, et al. Risk and management of bloodborne infections in health care workers. Clin Microbiol Rev 2000;13:385–407.
[15] McGrew CA. Blood-borne pathogens and sports. In: Fields KB, Fricker PA, editors. Medical problems in athletes. Oxford (UK): Blackwell Science; 1997. p. 64–9.
[16] Mast EE, Goodman RA, Bond WW, et al. Transmission of blood-borne pathogens during sports: risk and prevention. Ann Intern Med 1995;122:283–5.
[17] Brown LS, Drotman DP, Chu A, et al. Bleeding injuries in professional football. Estimating the risk for HIV transmission. Ann Intern Med 1995;122:271–4.
[18] Siebert DJ, Lindschau PB, Burrell CJ. Lack of evidence for significant hepatitis B transmission in Australian Rules footballers. Med J Aust 1995;162:312–3.
[19] Nattiv A, Puffer JC, Green GA. Lifestyles and health risks of collegiate athletes: a multi-center study. Clin J Sport Med 1997;7:262–72.
[20] Befeler AS, Di Bisceglie AM. Hepatitis B. Infect Dis Clin North Am 2000;14:617–32.

[21] Lok AS, McMahon BJ. Chronic hepatitis B. Hepatology 2001;34:1225–41.

[22] Aach RD, Stevens CD, Hollinger FB, et al. Hepatitis C virus infection in post-transfusion hepatitis. An analysis with first- and second-generation assays. N Engl J Med 1991;325: 1325–9.

[23] Alter HJ, Jett BW, Polito AJ, et al. Analysis of the role of hepatitis C virus in transfusion-associated hepatitis. In: Hollinger FB, Lemon SM, Margolis HS, editors. Viral hepatitis and liver disease. Baltimore(MD): Williams & Wilkins; 1991. p. 396–402.

[24] Koretz RL, Abbey H, Coleman E, et al. Non-A, non-B post-transfusion hepatitis: looking back in the second decade. Ann Intern Med 1993;119:110–5.

[25] Alter M. Epidemiology and disease burden of hepatitis B and C. Antivir Ther 1996;1:9–14.

[26] Morrison CL. Anabolic steroid users identified by needle and syringe exchange contact. Drug Alcohol Depend 1994;36:153–6.

[27] Aitken C, Delalande J, Stanton K. Pumping iron, risking infection? Drug Alcohol Depend 2002;65:303–8.

[28] Pediatrics Committee on Sports Medicine and Fitness. Human immunodeficiency virus and other blood-borne viral pathogens in the athletic setting. Pediatrics 1999;104;1400–3.

[29] Moyer LA, Mast EE, Alter MJ, et al. Hepatitis C: Part I. Routine serologic testing and diagnosis. Am Fam Physisian 1999;59:79–90.

[30] Powell DW, Abramson BZ, Baliant JA, et al. National Institutes of Health Consensus Development Conference Panel Statement: management of hepatitis C. Hepatology 1997;26(3 Suppl 1):2S–10S.

[31] Hoofnagle JH, Di Bisceglie AM. The treatment of chronic viral hepatitis. N Engl J Med 1997;336:347–56.

[32] Fried MW. Therapy of chronic viral hepatitis. Med Clin North Am 1996;80:957–72.

[33] Crampin AC, Lamagni TL, Hope VD, et al. The risk of infection with HIV and hepatitis B in individuals who inject steroids in England and Wales. Epidemiol Infect 1998;121(2): 381–6.

Clin Sports Med 26 (2007) 433–448

CLINICS IN SPORTS MEDICINE

ELSEVIER
SAUNDERS

Gastrointestinal Infections in the Athlete

Steven J. Karageanes, DO, FAOASM

Oakwood Sports Medicine, 9398 Lilley Road, Plymouth, MI 48170, USA

G astrointestinal (GI) infections can be a troublesome and debilitating illness to manage for sports medicine physicians. With the close proximity of athletes in locker rooms, living spaces, and accommodations when traveling, GI pathogens can rapidly spread throughout the team members and coaching staff.

In general, GI infections contribute significantly to the overall burden of human disease [1,2]. In 2001, a FoodNet surveillance system estimated that there are 76 million cases of food-borne disease each year [3]. These cases represent only a small portion of all enteric infections, the remainder of which may be transmitted by way of water consumption or person-to-person contact.

Most GI infections are self-limiting, but some cases can be fatal [1,4]. In the twentieth century, mortality rates from GI infections plummeted with the advent of disinfection of drinking water. For instance, in 1990, all infectious disease, including respiratory and GI, accounted for only 1.8% of deaths [1]; however, the proportion of Americans at risk for GI infections increases each year due compromised immune status or advancing age [1].

In addition, GI infection mortality is highest for the elderly and the young. In a study examining mortality rates from enteric disease from 1989 to 1996, the age groups most affected by viral enteric disease were patients older than 75 years, followed by patients younger than 5 years. The typical athlete fits into the two age groups that have the lowest mortality from GI infection (Box 1).

The high school and collegiate athlete have reasons to be wary of GI infections. The nature of their athletic activity sets them up for acute outbreaks of enteric disease. Two university campuses reported acute GI infection outbreaks that affected approximately 8% of the student body at large [5]. Most outbreaks occur in clusters, like in resident halls. In many cases, the source of infection cannot be identified [5].

E-mail address: drscoop@comcast.net

0278-5919/07/$ – see front matter
doi:10.1016/j.csm.2007.04.007

Box 1: The age groups with the highest rate of viral enteric disease mortality, from 1989 to 1996

>75 years old

<5 years old

55–64 years old

45–54 years old

35–44 years old

25–34 years old

5–24 years old

Data from Peterson CA, Calderon RL. Trends in enteric disease as a cause of death in the United States, 1989–1996. Am J Epidemiol 2003;157:58–65.

Other reasons for acute GI infections in the college or university setting include the following [5]:

Exposure to common sources of food, water, and environment

Person-to-person contact, particularly in athletics

Students who work as food handlers for income in campus dining facilities

Dormitory lifestyle, whereby students share basic elements such as bathrooms, living areas, and snack foods. This lifestyle includes athletic forums, like training rooms, locker rooms, and team meal facilities

Because of the ready access to student health care services, outbreaks on university campuses may be reported more frequently and efficiently than in the general population; however, the risk factors are undeniable.

Athletic competition, even one contest, provides enough contact to spread a GI pathogen. In particular, a 1998 GI infection outbreak among the University of North Carolina football team and staff started with turkey sandwiches in a catered box lunch [6]. Out of 108 players and staff, 54 developed an illness, with 43 having primary infections within 10 hours of consumption. Twenty-nine players developed the illness right before or during their game against the University of Florida. Eleven players on the Florida team developed the same GI infections, not from eating the same food, but from playing against the North Carolina team. The 11 players developed the illness, diagnosed as a form of Norwalk virus, within 48 hours of the game [6]. Other cases have had outbreaks in freshman dining halls, with 102 cases reported in a single day [7].

The National Collegiate Athletic Association does not mandate vaccinations for athletes because few have been shown effective. Vaccines exist for rotavirus, but it rarely affects athletes in the adolescent age range. Proper hygiene guidelines exist, and they have been shown to limit the spread of infection [1,4,5]. It falls on the sports medicine staff to enforce these guidelines and educate the athletes how and why these problems occur.

HISTORY

The predominant chief complaint in GI infections is diarrhea. A clinician should obtain a comprehensive medical history of the athlete whenever symptoms of the GI tract appear. Some important questions include the following [1]:

1. Symptoms—Diarrhea? If so, is it watery or bloody? Is there an appearance of oil or foamy soap? Explosive? Is there bloating, pain, cramping, nausea, vomiting, or constipation? Loss of appetite? Can the athlete ingest any nutrition?
2. Onset—How and when did the symptoms first appear? Frequent daily diarrhea? Intermittent cramping? How many days ago? Five or more days of symptoms may indicate more severe illness or a systemic illness with GI manifestations.
3. Provocative factors—Bloating or diarrhea after eating? Worse with solid foods, spicy foods, dairy products?
4. Medications—What medications has the athlete taken, including antibiotics? If not on antibiotics currently, was the athlete on them near the onset of symptoms?
5. Medical history—Recent hospitalizations? History of systemic disease? Is immune status compromised?
6. Dietary history—Recent consumption of fish (including sushi), meats (even fried meat), dairy products? Can the athlete hydrate properly?
7. Social history—Any travel out of the country or region? Any use of alcohol, tobacco, or illicit drugs? Any use of intravenous drugs? Recent living arrangements in close quarters? Any current roommate or family member with similar symptoms? Exposure to farm animals?
8. Sexual history—Any receptive anal intercourse or oral–anal sexual contact?
9. Review of systems—Fevers or chills? Palpitations? Joint pain? Ulcerations in the mouth? Rashes? Malaise or fatigue? Weight loss? Dry mouth? Changes in urination habits?

PHYSICAL EXAMINATION

Athletes may need a comprehensive physical examination to appropriately diagnose the ailment and to determine the need for more aggressive treatment. A careful examination should include the following:

Rectal examination for tenderness and for stool collection
Overall appearance, including mental status (ie, septic or toxic appearance)
Vital signs, including hypotension, high temperature
Postural changes in blood pressure and pulse
Skin turgor and mucous membrane examination
Abdominal examination for tenderness or peritoneal signs

LABORATORY AND IMAGING STUDIES

Multiple laboratory tests exist to aid in diagnosing the infectious pathogen causing gastroenteritis. Most diarrhea cases are self-limiting, so laboratory tests should not be done routinely. Rather, they should be used in severe cases or to help tailor the treatment in recalcitrant cases.

Laboratory studies commonly used to diagnose or rule out infectious causes include the following:

1. Fecal leukocyte determination—microscopic examination of stool samples prepared by methylene blue staining, used to look at inflammatory diarrheas. The sensitivity of this examination is 60%. The presence of fecal leukocytes supports the diagnosis of a bacterial cause of diarrhea in the context of the medical history. The Practice Parameters Committee of the American College of Gastroenterology recommends fecal leukocyte testing in patients who have moderate to severe diarrhea, although it is probably not helpful in patients who develop diarrhea while hospitalized [1].

2. Stool culture for enteric pathogens—this test should be ordered in patients who have severe dysentery, severe diarrhea, or stool that contains leukocytes. Most laboratories only process cultures for three organisms: *Shigella, Campylobacter,* and *Salmonella.* If high suspicion exists for other organisms, the laboratory should be notified immediately.

3. Stool culture for parasites—this test should be reserved for patients who have a high likelihood of parasitic infestation, such as patients who have AIDS and diarrhea, patients who have traveled internationally to endemic regions, or patients exposed to affected infants. Routine examination of stool for ova and parasites is not cost-effective in the workup of acute diarrhea. At least three stool specimens are needed to maximize chances of catching the parasites and ova in the stool [1].

4. *Clostridium difficile* toxin testing—this infection is seen in patients who have had previous hospitalization and have closed-community living arrangements, recent or remote antibiotic usage, and recent chemotherapy.

5. Flexible sigmoidoscopy with biopsy—endoscopy is rarely indicated in acute GI infections with diarrhea. Patients who have suspected *Clostridium difficile* infection may benefit from visualizing pseudomembranes caused by the pathogen.

Reasons for doing laboratory diagnostic studies include the following:

Grossly bloody stools
Profuse diarrhea with dehydration
Passage of more than six unformed stools per day or duration of illness longer than 48 hours
Fever (oral temperature >38.5°C)
Severe abdominal pain
Diarrhea in the immunocompromised or elderly

Imaging studies such as flexible sigmoidoscopy, colonoscopy, and contrast barium imaging are usually not indicated except for ruling out systemic disease such as inflammatory bowel disease or diverticulitis.

INFECTIOUS PATHOGENS

GI infections are divided into four categories: viral, parasitic, bacterial, and food-borne.

Viral

Noroviruses

Epidemiology. Noroviruses (formerly known as Norwalk-like viruses) are classified as a type of human calcivirus. They are the leading cause of acute, epidemic gastroenteritis in adults and older children in the United States [5] and worldwide [8]. Nearly all adults and most children have antibodies against the virus [8].

Transmission. Transmission is by the fecal–oral route. Most outbreaks come from fecal contamination of water or food by an infected handler. Food was implicated in 39% of norovirus cases reported to the Centers for Disease Control and Prevention between 1996 and 2000 [9]. Other routes are postulated but not proven.

Pathogenesis. There are no animal models, only studies done on human volunteers. After infection of the virus, small lesions in the small intestine appear, showing villus shortening, crypt hyperplasia, and infiltration of the lamina propria by polymorphonuclear cells and lymphocytes [10]. The lesions persist after symptoms resolve, causing malabsorption of carbohydrates and fats [10].

History.

> Viral incubation: 12 to 48 hours
> Illness duration: 12 to 60 hours
> Typical vectors of transmission: water or food, usually shellfish
> Contagious period: during onset of symptoms until 48 hours after diarrhea resolves
> Immunity: short-term (14 weeks)

Symptoms. Symptoms include nausea, vomiting, abdominal cramping, constitutional symptoms, and diarrhea. It should be noted that in children, vomiting is more common than diarrhea; conversely, adults have more diarrhea than vomiting.

Laboratory detection. Southern blot analysis based on polymerase chain reaction amplification has led to the development of immunoassays to identify the virus in stool; however, they are not widely used or available [10].

Treatment. The infection is self-limited, so only rehydration for support may be indicated. With the average athlete, hospitalization is rarely needed.

Prevention. Prevention includes frequent hand washing, especially after practices, games, and handling athletic clothing; avoiding contact with food by sick or infected food handlers; and practicing good personal hygiene. Vaccines are being developed but are not yet available.

Rotavirus. Rotavirus infections are rarely seen past age 3 years; the incidence peaks in children from age 4 months to 23 months. Rotavirus infection is not often seen in the athletic setting, although parents of infected young children have been known to exhibit subacute symptoms of rotavirus [10].

Parasitic
Giardia

Epidemiology. *Giardia* is a protozoan that primarily infects the upper small intestine. Its spread is worldwide, and children are affected more than adults. Regions with poor sanitation or poor potty training in day care facilities have a higher risk of carrying giardiasis. The prevalence of stool positivity in different areas may range between 1% and 30%, depending on the area and region.

Transmission. Person-to-person, hand-to-mouth contact is the most common route. Other sources include anal intercourse and fecally contaminated food and water.

History.

> Bacterial incubation: 3 to 25 days or longer; median 7 to 10 days
> Typical vectors of transmission: contaminated food and water
> Contagious period: during whole illness, even months
> Immunity: short-term (14 weeks)

Symptoms. There are various manifestations of the infection:

1. Asymptomatic yet infected
2. Acute, self-limiting diarrhea
3. Intestinal effects: chronic diarrhea; malabsorption (of fats and fat-soluble vitamins); steatorrhea; abdominal cramps; frequent loose and pale, greasy stools; fatigue; bloating; and weight loss

In a few cases, reactive arthritis and duodenal and jejunal mucosal cell damage can occur.

Laboratory detection. Identification of cysts or trophozoites in feces under microscopy is most effective. At least three negative stool samples must be obtained to rule out giardiasis. Enzyme-linked immunosorbent assay or direct fluorescent antibody methods to detect antigens in the stool are available.

Treatment.

> Metronidazole, 250 mg po TID for 5 to 7 days (children, 15 mg/kg/day divided TID for 5 days)
> Tinidazole, 2 g in a single dose (children, 50–75 mg/kg)

Prevention.

> Educate athletes' families, day care professionals, and people working or living in institutions on hygiene and hand washing.
> Use water filtration.
> Dispose of feces in a hygienic and sanitary manner.
> Boil emergency water supplies. Use 0.1 to 0.2 mL (2–4 drops) of household bleach or 0.5 mL of 2% tincture of iodine per liter for 20 minutes, more if the water is cold.
> Disinfect soiled clothes, towels, jerseys, or practice uniforms.

Entamoeba histolytica

Epidemiology. *Entamoeba histolytica* is a pathogenic species capable of causing disease such as colitis or liver abscess in humans [11]. There are numerous distinct species within the genus *Entamoeba*, but most do not cause disease in humans. Some estimate that 10% of the world's population is infected with *Entamoeba histolytica* or *Entamoeba dispar*, of which less than 10% manifest disease [11].

Pathogenesis. *Entamoeba histolytica* exists in one of two forms—a cyst or a trophozoite. Infection is generally through fecal–oral spread with ingestion of the cyst form, which is resistant to killing by the low pH of the stomach [12]. The cysts split to form trophozoites, which go to the large intestine. Production of proteolytic enzymes allows the trophozoite to disrupt tissue planes and invade the colonic epithelium. These enzymes can lyse neutrophils through a contact-dependent mechanism, causing local tissue damage but protecting the trophozoite.

Laboratory detection. Detection is by way of demonstration of cysts or trophozoites in the stool or by examination of biopsy specimens of mucosal tissue. Testing using monoclonal antibodies and polymerase chain reaction is emerging, which may help differentiate *Entamoeba histolytica* and *Entamoeba dispar* [13].

Symptoms. Acute amebic colitis usually presents with several weeks of lower abdominal pain and diarrhea with frequent loose to watery stools containing blood and mucus [12]. Most patients are afebrile. Significant volume depletion is uncommon. Chronic amebic colitis is characterized by low-grade inflammation resulting in intermittent bloody diarrhea and abdominal pain over a period of months to years. It is often difficult to distinguish chronic disease from inflammatory bowel disease [14].

Amebic liver abscess is the most common extraintestinal manifestation of amebiasis [14]. Less than 50% of patients have an enlarged liver, and diarrhea is found in less than one third of patients. Patients may note right-upper-quadrant pain that is dull or pleuritic in nature, referring to the right shoulder. Acute patients typically manifest fever, whereas subacute cases (longer than 2 weeks) have fever in less than half of the cases. Respiratory symptoms such as cough can occur even in the absence of pulmonary disease and may be the only complaint. In the subacute setting, weight loss is common.

Other symptoms or manifestations include change in mental status, focal neurologic deficits, congestive heart failure, and genitourinary painful ulcers with profuse discharge [14].

Treatment.

> Treatment requires the elimination of the trophozoite form from the intestine or extraintestinal sites, and the elimination of cysts from the intestine [14]
> Metronidazole (agent of choice), 750 mg three times daily for 5 to 10 days orally or intravenously for amebiasis and amebic liver abscess
> Tetracycline or erythromycin—milder cases of colitis

Iodoquinol (diiodohydroxyquin)—preferred luminal agent
    20 days of therapy
    May interfere with thyroid function tests and should be avoided in patients
        allergic to iodine
Paromomycin—luminal agent

Bacterial

Campylobacter

Epidemiology. *Campylobacter* is the most common cause of bacterial gastroenteritis in the world. England and Wales report an average of 50,000 cases per year, and the trend is not declining [15]. *Campylobacter* is responsible for 15% of all traveler's diarrhea from Asia.

Transmission. Transmission is by the fecal–oral route. Most outbreaks come from fecal contamination of water or food (most often chicken) by an infected handler [4]. Other routes are postulated but not proven.

Pathogenesis. *Campylobacter jejuni* and, less commonly, *Campylobacter coli* are the main bacterial agents causing diarrhea through toxin elaboration and mucosal invasion [4]. There are over 20 other biotypes of *Campylobacter*. Most infections occur in immunocompromised hosts.

History.

Duration: symptoms occur 2 to 5 days after exposure and can last from 24 hours to 1 week
Contagious period: from onset of symptoms until 48 hours after diarrhea resolved
Immunity: short-term (14 weeks).

Symptoms. Symptoms include diarrhea (frequently with bloody stools), abdominal pain, malaise, fever, and nausea with or without vomiting. Gross or occult blood with mucus and white blood cells is often present in liquid stools. Cases may mimic acute appendicitis or inflammatory bowel disease. Infection can less commonly manifest as a typhoid-like syndrome, meningeal syndrome, or febrile convulsions [16].

Laboratory detection. Detection is by way of isolation of the organisms from stools using selective media, reduced oxygen tension, and incubation at 43°C (109.4°F). Microscopy can visualize motile organisms that are curved, spiral, or S-shaped rods.

Treatment. Many infections are asymptomatic and occasionally self-limited. With the average athlete, hospitalization is rarely needed.

Prevention. Prevention includes frequent hand washing, especially after practices, games, and handling athletic clothing; avoiding contact with food by sick or infected food handlers; and practicing good personal hygiene. Vaccines are being developed but are not yet available.

Enterohemorrhagic Escherichia coli

Epidemiology. Enterohemorrhagic *Escherichia coli* (EHEC) is the most common cause of infectious bloody diarrhea [4]. Subtype O157:H7 is well known as a cause of hemorrhagic colitis and may be associated with hemolytic uremic syndrome.

Pathogenesis. EHEC is not invasive, but its cytotoxin causes endothelial damage, microangiopathic hemolysis, and renal damage. The toxin produced by EHEC is closely related to that produced by *Shigella* and is called Shiga toxin. The enteropathogenic *Escherichia coli* strains lack Shiga toxin production and cause nonspecific diarrhea in infants in less-developed countries [17].

There are five other subtypes of *Escherichia coli* that cause enteric disease. One such strain is enterotoxigenic *Escherichia coli* (ETEC). This infection is seen in developed countries that have poor water sanitation and drinking-water treatment facilities. ETEC is transmitted by contaminated, improperly treated drinking water, and its incidence peaks in the warm, wet seasons that favor environmental bacterial replication.

Transmission. Transmission is by the fecal–oral route, primarily through ingesting contaminated undercooked ground beef, unpasteurized apple juice, milk, lettuce, or venison. Secondary infections can be contracted from household contacts or children and personnel in day care centers [4].

Laboratory detection. Detection is by way of toxin testing of stool with Shiga toxin–based assays or stool culture on sorbitol-MacConkey agar, with subsequent serotyping.

Onset. Symptom onset usually occurs 7 to 10 days after the consumption of contaminated meat or water.

Symptoms. Symptoms include moderate to severe diarrhea (10–12 liquid stools/day), which may progress to bloody diarrhea. Severe cramping, abdominal pain, nausea, and vomiting are seen in approximately two thirds of patients. Examination can reveal abdominal distention, generalized or focal right-lower-quadrant tenderness, and bloody stool on rectal examination.

Course. About 5% to 10% of cases develop hemolytic uremic syndrome, which is diagnosed about 5 to 6 days after onset of diarrhea. Of those patients, up to 5% die acutely, 5% develop end-stage renal disease, and up to 30% have long-term sequelae such as proteinuria. Neurologic manifestations of thrombotic thrombocytopenic purpura, such as myoclonic jerking and confusion, can also occur.

Treatment.

> Supportive care is indicated based on the specific manifestations. The course is self-limiting, although 5% may require hospitalization. Particular attention to fluid status is essential to limit renal and vascular complications.
> Antibiotics have not been shown to be effective and may increase the risk of hemolytic uremic syndrome [4].

Salmonella

Epidemiology. There are two classes of *Salmonella*: typhoid (*Salmonella typhi and Salmonella paratyphi*) and nontyphoid (*Salmonella enteriditis and Salmonella typhimurium*). Typhoid fever is a systemic disease that involves a prolonged febrile illness, splenomegaly, delirium, and abdominal pain but few GI-specific manifestations. Nontyphoid *Salmonella*, however, is the leading cause of food poisoning in the United States. Infections are seen more in the summer and fall months and classically seen in animal products such as poultry, beef, milk, and eggs.

Transmission. Transmission is by the fecal–oral route, with consumption of contaminated animal products being the main cause of salmonellosis.

Laboratory detection. Blood cultures are positive in only 5% to 10% of cases.

Course. Illness lasts less than 7 days and is normally self-limiting.

Symptoms. Patients suffer from fever, chills, nausea, vomiting, diarrhea, and abdominal cramping. Bloody stools are rarely seen.

Treatment. Treatment consists of supportive care, with monitoring and support of fluid status. Antibiotic use is indicated only when the patient is very young or old and has focal infections (eg, abscesses or osteomyelitis), immunodeficiency, or signs of sepsis. The drug of choice is trimethoprim-sulfamethoxazole for 5 to 7 days or a third-generation cephalosporin.

Shigella

Epidemiology. *Shigella* is the second most common food-borne disease in the United States and one of the most common causes of dysentery. It is a facultative anaerobic, gram-negative bacilli closely related to *Escherichia coli*. Shigellosis causes an estimated 600,000 deaths per year. Two thirds of the cases and most of the deaths are in children younger than 10 years. Outbreaks occur under conditions of crowding and where personal hygiene is poor. Shigellosis is endemic in tropical and temperate climates.

Two classes of *Shigella* organisms exist, with four serotypes overall: watery (*Shigella sonnei, Shigella boydii*) or dysenteric (*Shigella dysenteriae, Shigella flexneri*). The prevalence of *Shigella* is cyclic, with replacement of the predominant strain approximately every 20 years [17]. Virulence differs between the dysenteric and watery species. *Shigella dysenteriae* infections can be fatal in up to 20% of hospitalized cases, whereas hosts who have *Shigella sonnei* have short clinical courses and almost no fatalities (except in immunocompromised hosts).

Pathogenesis. Shigellosis causes water diarrhea by superficial mucosal invasion of the organisms and luminal bacterial replication. The organisms soon migrate into the colon, where mucosal sloughing occurs from Shiga toxin production or mucosal invasion. The sloughing causes an acute inflammatory response, tenesmus, and small-volume bloody or mucoid stools. In prolonged cases, shigellosis can mimic ulcerative colitis.

Laboratory detection. Definitive diagnosis requires microbiologic isolation and identification of *Shigella* species or molecular evidence of infection from feces or rectal swabs. The appropriate media must be used and samples processed quickly because the organisms are viable for only a short time outside the host [15]. Infection is usually associated with large numbers of fecal leukocytes detected through microscopic examination of stool mucus stained with methylene blue or Gram stain.

Imaging. Colonoscopy may be done to rule out inflammatory bowel disease, especially if laboratory detection is difficult. The appearance of pseudomembranes, colonic mucosal sloughing, and lumenal inflammation mimics ulcerative colitis.

Onset. Shigellosis has 1- to 3-day incubation period; however, incubation can be up to a week with *Shigella dysenteriae.* Cases are self-limiting, with the average length being 4 to 7 days [4,17].

Symptoms. When *Shigella* invades the small intestine early on, the patient suffers from acute, watery diarrhea, fever, and abdominal pain. Patients may become toxemic, and fever may reach as high as 104°F. When the organisms migrate into the large intestine, pain is in lower abdominal quadrants, and fever may persist. Stools become dysenteric, consisting of a mixture of neutrophils, blood, mucus, and debris. Rectal pruritis and pain is common [4,17].

Transmission. Transmission is by the fecal–oral route from contaminated food or water, usually from a symptomatic individual or short-term carrier. *Shigella* is the only bacterial enteric pathogen that can be transmitted person to person because it transverses the gastric acid barrier [4].

Treatment.

> Supportive therapy is indicated because the disease is self-limiting. Fluid and electrolytes should be replaced with any significant watery diarrheal condition.
>
> Antimicrobials are used to shorten the course and limit potential for outbreak. Trimethoprim-sulfamethoxazole or fluoroquinolones for 3 days are preferred [17].
>
> Resistance against multidrug regimens is rising, even against fluoroquinolones, so specific sensitivities may be needed.
>
> Antimotility drugs (eg, loperamide) must not be used in children.

Prevention. As with most infectious enteric pathogens, *Shigella* is best controlled by proper hygiene, especially in cramped athletic team settings. Proper hygiene includes simple hand washing with soap and water. Outbreaks in the United States are rare, but team travel to endemic locations is not unusual. The medical staff should be cognizant of this and take the appropriate precautions with respect to food, water, and hygiene. Training staff may need to observe hand washing when the team is in an endemic region.

Due to its propensity for large outbreaks, *Shigella* infection cases should be reported to the proper authorities, and the source should be determined and isolated. Anyone with a known *Shigella* infection should not be employed to touch or handle food or children in day care settings until that person has two *Shigella*-free successive fecal samples or rectal swabs, collected 24 or more hours apart, but not sooner than 48 hours after stopping antimicrobials [17].

Food-Borne

Food-borne illnesses from infectious agents are not necessarily infections causing symptoms of gastroenteritis. In general, food-borne illness comes from (1) toxins in the food from bacterial growth; (2) bacterial, viral, or parasitic infections (covered earlier in this article); and (3) toxins produced by harmful algal species (ciguatera fish poisoning or paralytic, neurotoxic, diarrheic, or amnesic shellfish poisoning) or present in specific species (puffer fish, azaspiracids). Table 1 shows the common sources of food-borne illnesses.

Food contaminated with toxins from bacteria can cause severe illness, but not by infestation. Rather, the GI tract reacts to the toxin when ingested. It may be the most common cause of gastroenteritis, but many cases go unreported.

Organisms

The most common pathogens are listed in Table 2. Most of these organisms do not affect the typical American athlete (due to age, immune status, or region); however, because athletic teams occasionally travel to tournaments in other countries, the list is complete for reference.

Symptoms

Cases can be mild or severe, depending on the agent. Cruise ships have been high-profile examples of outbreaks of gastroenteritis due to food contamination from toxin and infection [18].

Table 1
Examples of principal bacterial causes of food poisoning

Bacterial species	Common foods that can be contaminated
Bacillus cereus	Cooked rice, meat
Campylobacter species	Poultry, unpasteurized milk
Clostridium botulinum	Fish, meat
Clostridium perfringens	Cooked meat, poultry
Escherichia coli	Meat, raw milk
Listeria monocytogenes	Pâté, soft cheese
Salmonellae	Meat, poultry, eggs
Shigella species	Eggs, salad
Staphylococcus aureus	Ham, poultry, dairy products
Yersinia enterocolitica	Milk, poultry

Data from Gibson GR, McCartney AL, Rastall RA. Prebiotics and resistance to gastrointestinal infections. Brit J Nutr 2005;93(Suppl 1):S31–4.

Table 2
Common pathogens related to gastroenteritis from food poisoning, including common clinical syndrome and pathogenic mechanism of the pathogen

Organism	Clinical syndrome	Pathogenic mechanism
Salmonella serotypes	Dysentery	Mucosal invasion
Salmonella serotype Typhi	Enteric fever	Penetration, spread
Shigella spp	Dysentery	Mucosal invasion, cytotoxin
Shigella dysenteriae (Shiga)	Dysentery	Mucosal invasion, cytotoxin
Campylobacter jejuni	Dysentery	Unknown
Escherichia coli (EIEC)	Dysentery	Mucosal invasion
Escherichia coli (ETEC)	Dysentery	Enterotoxin(s)
Escherichia coli (EHEC)	Watery diarrhea	Cytotoxin
Escherichia E coli (EPEC)	Watery diarrhea	Adherence
Vibrio cholerae	Watery diarrhea	Enterotoxin
Vibrio parahaemolyticus	Watery diarrhea	Unknown
Yersinia enterocolitica	Enteric fever	Penetration, spread
Clostridium difficile	Dysentery	Cytotoxin, enterotoxin
Clostridium perfringens	Watery diarrhea	Enterotoxin
Bacillus cereus	Watery diarrhea	Enterotoxin
Rotavirus	Watery diarrhea	Mucosal destruction
Caliciviruses	Watery diarrhea	Mucosal destruction
Giardia lamblia	Watery diarrhea	Mucosal irritation
Entamoeba histolytica	Dysentery	Mucosal invasion
Cryptosporidium	Watery diarrhea	Possibly toxin

Abbreviations: EIEC, enteroinvasive *Escherichia coli*; EPEC, enteropathogenic *Escherichia coli*.
From Ryan KJ. Enteric infections and food poisoning. In: Ryan KJ, Ray CG, editors. Sherris medical microbiology. 4th edition. New York: McGraw Hill; 2004. p. 203; with permission.

Onset
Symptom onset usually occurs a short time after consumption of the affected food, from a few days to even a few weeks.

Prevention
Prevention depends on educating food handlers about proper practices in cooking and storage of food and in personal hygiene. The World Health Organization established the five keys for safer food to help curb the number of outbreaks (Box 2) [19].

Much of the difficulty in preventing food-borne illnesses lies in the differences in culture, technology, and resources between developed and underdeveloped countries. Methods of food preparation, hygiene, waste management, and water treatment differ, even among developed countries. Some countries fertilize with human excreta, which increases risk of transmission.

When traveling to regions of endemic food-borne disease, athletes and staff should follow the following guidelines:

Avoid drinking tap water, noncarbonated bottled water, unpasteurized milk, and iced drinks (including alcoholic drinks).
Only eat food served piping hot.
Avoid raw vegetables and fruits that cannot be peeled.

Box 2: Five keys for safer food

Keep clean

Separate raw and cooked

Cook thoroughly

Keep food at safe temperatures

Use safe water and raw materials

Only drink water treated by boiling at 100°C for 5 to 10 minutes, halogenation with iodine or chlorine, or filtration by sediment filtration or resin contact devices.

Avoid food that requires elaborate preparation.

Avoid foods containing dairy products.

Prebiotics

Research exists supporting the use of prebiotics to reduce pathogenesis of the GI tract [19–23]. By fortifying the gut flora and improving resistance against colonization, prebiotics can be a dietary intervention to curb the number of outbreaks of toxic and invasive viral and bacterial gastroenteritis [19]. The gut flora consists of lactobacilli and bifidobacteria that can exist in environments that most pathologic organisms cannot. The suggested mechanisms of how the gut flora resists colonization are listed in Box 3 [19].

Prophylaxis

In general, prophylactic antibiotics and bismuth sulfate are not standard recommendations for travelers, despite proven efficacy in both regimens [4]. Arguments exist on both sides whether all travelers should use prophylaxis. The biggest deterrent is the potential for side effects, such as Stevens-Johnson

Box 3: Proposed mechanisms of resistance of gut flora to pathogen colonization of the gastrointestinal tract

Metabolic end products, such as acids, excreted by gut flora may lower the gut pH, in a microniche, to levels below those at which pathogens are able to effectively compete

Direct antagonism through natural antimicrobial excretion (lactic acid bacteria produce inhibitory peptides)

Competitive effects from occupation of normal colonization sites

Competition for nutrients, which may be limiting

Enhancement of the immune system

Data from Gibson GR, McCartney AL, Rastall RA. Prebiotics and resistance to gastrointestinal infections. Brit J Nutr 2005;93(Suppl 1):S32–3.

Box 4: Prophylactic treatment against traveler's diarrhea

Bismuth subsalicylate: two tablets with meals and at bedtime (eight tablets a day)

Fluoroquinolones: one tablet once a day

    Ciprofloxacin, 500 mg (1st choice)

    Norfloxacin, 400 mg

    Ofloxacin, 300 mg

From Lung EE. Acute diarrheal diseases. In: Friedman SL, McQuad KR, Grendell JH, et al, editors. Current diagnosis and treatment in gastroenterology. 2nd edition. New York: McGraw-Hill, Inc.; 2003. p. 154–5; with permission.

---

syndrome and anaphylaxis [24]. The following groups of travelers, however, should be considered for chemoprophylaxis [4,24]:

    Those who cannot tolerate inactivity (athlete, politician, performing artist)

    Those who have underlying medical disorders in whom diarrhea would be poorly tolerated

    Those who have repeated bouts of traveler's diarrhea and known poor compliance with general food and water precautions

The author therefore recommends that athletes traveling to regions where enteric pathogens are endemic use chemoprophylaxis to lower risk of gastroenteritis from food-borne pathogens. Treatment regimens are found in Box 4 [4].

Regimens should be started on the day of arrival in the country and continued for 1 to 2 days after leaving. Medication should not be continued after 3 weeks [25].

References

[1] Peterson CA, Calderon RL. Trends in enteric disease as a cause of death in the United States, 1989–1996. Am J Epidemiol 2003;157:58–65.

[2] Centers for Disease Control and Prevention. Preliminary FoodNet data on the incidence of foodborne illnesses—selected sites, United States, 2001. MMWR Morb Mortal Wkly Rep 2002;51:325–9.

[3] Lung EE. Acute diarrheal diseases. In: Friedman SL, McQuad KR, Grendell JH, et al, editors. Current diagnosis and treatment in gastroenterology. 2nd edition. New York: McGraw-Hill, Inc.; 2003. p. 414–8.

[4] Moe CL, Christmas WA, Echols LJ, et al. Outbreaks of acute gastroenteritis associated with Norwalk-like viruses in campus settings. J Am Coll Health 2001;50(2):57–66.

[5] Becker KM, Moe CL, Southwick KL, et al. Transmission of Norwalk virus during a football game. N Engl J Med 2000;343:1223–7.

[6] Kilgore PE, Belay ED, Hamlin DM, et al. A university outbreak of gastroenteritis due to a small round-structured virus: application of molecular diagnostics to identify the etiologic agent and patterns of transmission. J Infect Dis 2000;181:1467–70.

[7] Khetsurian N, Parashar UD. Enteric viral infections. In: Dale DC, editor. Infectious diseases: the clinician's guide to diagnosis, treatment, and prevention. Teton Data Systems; 2006. Available at: http://online.statref.com/document.aspx?fxid=65&;docid=281. Accessed October 1, 2006.

[8] Dippold L, Lee R, Selman C, et al. A gastroenteritis outbreak due to norovirus associate with a Colorado hotel. J Environ Health 2003;66(5):13–7.

[9] Schreiber DS, Blacklow NR, Trier JS. The mucosal lesion of the proximal small intestine in acute infectious nonbacterial gastroenteritis. N Engl J Med 1973;288:1318–23.

[10] Reed SL. Amebiasis: an update. Clin Infect Dis 1992;14(5):1161–2.

[11] Warhurst DC. Diagnosis of amebic infection. In: Gillespie SH, Hawkey PM, editors. Medical parasitology, a practical approach. New York: Oxford University Press; 1995. p. 131–4.

[12] Reed SL, Wessel DW, Davis CE. *Entamoeba histolytica* infection and AIDS. Am J Med 1991;90:269–71.

[13] Fox CR, Sande MA. Pathogenic amebas. Wilson WR, Sande MA. Current diagnosis and treatment in infectious diseases. New York: Lange Medical Books/McGraw-Hill, 2001. p. 704–8.

[14] Evans MR, Ribiero CD, Salmon RL. Hazards of healthy living: bottled water and salad vegetables as risk factors for *Campylobacter* infection. Emerg Infect Dis 2003;9(10):1219–25.

[15] Robins-Browe RM, Bordun AM, Tauschek M, et al. *Escherichia coli* and community-acquired gastroenteritis, Melbourne, Australia. Emerg Infect Dis 2004;10(10):1797–805.

[16] Bren L. Cruising with confidence. FDA Consum 2003;37(3):34–5.

[17] Procop GW, Cockerill F. Enteritis caused by *Escherichia coli & Shigella & Salmonella* species. Wilson WR, Sande MA, editors. Current diagnosis and treatment in infectious diseases. New York: McGraw-Hill companies, 2001. p. 483–6

[18] World Health Organization. Prevention of foodborne disease: five keys to safer food, 2006. Available at: http://www.who.int/foodsafety/consumer/5keys/en/index2.html. Accessed October 10, 2006.

[19] Buddington KK, Danohoo JB, Buddington RK. Dietary oligofructose and inulin protect mice from enteric and systemic pathogens and tumour inducers. J Nutr 2002;132:472–7.

[20] Cummings JH, Christie S, Cole TJ. A study of fructooligosaccharides in the prevention of travellers' diarrhoea. Aliment Pharmacol Ther 2001;15:1139–45.

[21] Meyer DP, Tungland BC, Causey JL, et al. The immune effects of inulin in vitro and in vivo. Agro-Food Ind Hi Technol 2000;11:18–20.

[22] Kleessen B, Sykura B, Zunft H-J, et al. Effects of inulin and lactose on fecal microflora, microbial activity and bowel habit in elderly constipated persons. American Journal of Clinical Nutrition 1997;65:1397–402.

[23] Asahara T, Nomoto K, Shimizu K, et al. Increased resistance of mice to *Salmonella enlerilica* serovar Typhy-murium infection by synbiotic administration of bifidobacteria and transgalactosylated-oligosaccharides. J Appl Microbiol 2001;91:985–96.

[24] DuPont HL. Travellers' diarrhea: contemporary approaches to therapy and prevention. Drugs 2006;66(3):303–14.

[25] Ryan KJ. Enteric infections and food poisoning. Ryan KJ, Ray CG, editors. Sherris medical microbiology. 4th edition. New York: McGraw Hill, 2004. p. 387–92.

Clin Sports Med 26 (2007) 449–471

CLINICS IN SPORTS MEDICINE

ELSEVIER
SAUNDERS

Infectious Disease and the Collegiate Athlete

Robert G. Hosey, MD[a],*, Richard E. Rodenberg, MD[b]

[a]Department of Family and Community Medicine, Department of Orthopaedics,
Primary Care Sports Medicine Fellowship, University of Kentucky Chandler Medical Center,
K 433 Kentucky Clinic, 740 S. Limestone, Lexington, KY 40536, USA
[b]Grant Medical Center, 111 S. Grant Ave., Columbus, OH 43215, USA

A thletes, especially those at or above the collegiate level are subjected to significant travel, group meetings, and close living quarters, which may increase risk of exposure to infectious agents. In addition, there is some evidence to indicate that athletes tend to be risk takers, which may increase their likelihood of contracting certain types of infectious disease, most notably sexually transmitted diseases (STDs). As a result, infectious diseases in collegiate athletes account for a large percentage of encounters with the team physician. It is fortunate that most of these illnesses are accompanied by only mildly irritating symptoms and are generally short lived. In some cases, however, serious physical complications and difficult return-to-play decisions may arise.

INFECTIOUS MONONUCLEOSIS

Infectious mononucleosis (IM) is a common medical condition caused by Epstein-Barr virus (EBV). IM cases are encountered on a regular basis in collegiate athletes each year. Acute illness classically presents as a triad of fever, tonsillar pharyngitis, and lymphadenopathy. The clinical course is often variable, with a wide range of symptom severity. The potential for complications, including splenic rupture, can make return-to-activity decisions a difficult one for sports medicine physicians.

Epidemiology

EBV is a DNA herpesvirus that enters the squamous epithelial cells and is transmitted person to person by way of oropharyngeal secretions. As a result, it is often referred to as the "kissing disease." EBV has also been isolated from epithelial cells of the cervix and in semen and may be transmitted by blood transfusion [1]. The prevalence of IM in the general population is 45 cases in every 100,000 people. Peak incidence occurs in the 15- to 25-year-old age group. Approximately 30% to 50% of students commencing college remain

*Corresponding author. E-mail address: rhosey@email.uky.edu (R.G. Hosey).

0278-5919/07/$ – see front matter
doi:10.1016/j.csm.2007.04.005
sportsmed.theclinics.com

susceptible to acute infection, with 1% to 3% of the general student population acquiring the disease each year. Therefore, the rate of infection in this population approaches 15% [2]. In universities with large athletic populations, this could potentially translate to greater than 10 symptomatic cases of IM annually.

Individuals infected with EBV have variable clinical manifestations. Although 50% to 70% of adolescents and young adults experience significant clinical symptoms, less than 10% of infected children develop symptoms. The development of symptomatic IM in adults older than 35 years is uncommon, which may be due, in part, to the high likelihood of prior exposure (and subclinical disease), because nearly 95% of adults eventually develop antibodies to EBV.

Clinical Symptoms

The onset of clinical symptoms associated with EBV infection is often several weeks after exposure due to the extremely long incubation period, which ranges from 30 to 50 days. As a result, source identification is difficult. The commencement of symptomatic disease is preceded by an intense T cell–mediated response typically manifested by a 3- to 5-day prodromal period of symptoms consisting of headache, malaise, and myalgias. The prodromal symptoms herald the onset of the classic triad of fever, pharyngitis, and cervical lymphadenopathy (posterior nodes > anterior). Axillary and inguinal nodes can also be involved. Fatigue, palatal petechiae, and rash may also be present [3]. Associated splenic enlargement results from lymphocytic infiltration of the spleen and may cause vague abdominal discomfort. Hepatomegaly may occasionally occur, whereas jaundice is rarely encountered. There is a wide spectrum of symptom severity and longevity, but in most cases, resolution of clinical diseased occurs within 4 to 8 weeks.

Diagnosis

The diagnosis of IM remains predominately a clinical diagnosis. Laboratory tests are often used to help confirm clinical suspicion. An elevated white blood cell count in the range of 12,000 to 18,000 with greater than 50% lymphocytes and at least 10% atypical lymphocytes on the peripheral smear is consistent with IM diagnosis. The Monospot test, which tests for the presence of heterophile antibodies in the patient's serum, may be used as confirmatory test. Although it is relatively specific, its sensitivity varies, having false negative rates approaching 25% during the first week of illness and falling to 5% by the third week [4]. The use of heterophile antibody tests are classically unreliable in pediatric populations (age <10 years) in whom it is likely to detect less than half of EBV infections. In instances in which there is a strong clinical suspicion of IM and the Monospot test is negative, EBV titers should be measured. Immunoglobulin (Ig)G and IgM antibodies to viral capsule antigen are highly sensitive and specific for diagnosing IM. The continued absence of such antibodies to viral capsule antigen on repeat testing warrants consideration of alternative diagnoses. Similarly, the presence of antibodies to EBV nuclear antigen likely signifies prior and not acute infection because these antibodies typically develop later in the clinical course and are present indefinitely.

Complications

For most patients who have acute IM, symptoms are moderate in severity, and recovery is uneventful. Despite this fact, several potentially severe complications have been associated with IM, including Guillain-Barré syndrome, meningitis, neuritis, hemolytic uremic syndrome, disseminated intravascular coagulation, and aplastic anemia. In addition, obstruction from severe tonsillar enlargement can lead to acute respiratory compromise. In these instances, hospitalization and advanced airway management strategies may be necessary.

Prolonged fatigue is likely the most widely encountered complication of IM. For athletes, coaches, trainers, and sports practitioners, it is arguably the most frustrating aspect to deal with. Duration of symptoms in athletes is wide ranging, mirroring that of the general population. There is, however, some evidence to suggest that it takes up to 3 months for athletes to return to preillness level of activity [5]. Counseling the athlete and coaches during this rather lengthy convalescent time may prove essential to remove unreal expectations regarding performance.

Perhaps the most widely feared and well-known complication of acute IM is splenic rupture. It has been reported to occur in approximately 0.1% to 0.2% of IM cases [6]. A case series documenting splenic rupture in collegiate athletes indicated IM as an associated factor in over one third of the reported cases [7]. The current prevailing theory suggests that lymphocytic infiltration of the spleen distorts the normal anatomy and weakens the supporting structures, resulting in increased splenic fragility. Although the main concern is about a traumatic event leading to rupture in these individuals, it is just as likely for the spleen to rupture without identifiable trauma in these patients [2]. In athletes who have IM, splenic rupture has predominately been documented to occur in the first 3 weeks of the illness [2]; however, there are case reports of splenic rupture as long as 7 weeks from the onset of clinical symptoms [8]. This variability in presentation inevitably raises questions and concerns regarding athletes' safe return to participation.

Treatment

The mainstay of treatment for acute IM cases involves measures aimed at symptom relief and supportive care. Rest, fever control, and maintaining hydration status are important. Painful pharyngitis may be improved by use of topical anesthetics, acetaminophen, or both. Although no controlled studies have evaluated the efficacy of corticosteroids in limiting duration of symptoms or preventing complications associated with IM, these medications are often used. In general, use of corticosteroids should be limited to individuals who have severe hepatitis, myocarditis, hemolytic uremic syndrome, and neurologic complications. In addition, they may be recommended for patients at risk of airway obstruction secondary to significant enlargement of tonsils and adenoids.

Diagnostic Imaging

Historically, physicians have used the presence of an enlarged spleen associated with acute IM as an important factor in the decision to allow an athlete to safely resume physical activity. Because the ability to detect the presence of an enlarged spleen by physical examination alone has poor sensitivity and specificity, advanced radiographic procedures are often used in these cases [9].

CT scans and ultrasounds provide quality imaging of the spleen with the ability to accurately assess splenic dimensions. Although CT offers better anatomic detail, sonography is readily available, is less expensive, and eliminates significant radiation exposure. Literature standards define the upper limits of normal splenic length as 12 to 14 cm in adults [10–12]. There may be some problems, however, in trying to apply normative values to the general population as a whole or to specific populations such as athletes. The problem arises because the populations on which these values were defined were often heterogeneous and the individual sample sizes within specific age groups were small [13–19].

A recent study of 631 collegiate athletes demonstrated considerable variability of normal splenic size among the athletes (average spleen length 10.65 cm; range 5.59–17.06 cm). In this study, spleen size correlated with height and weight but varied significantly between sexes and among races. Slightly more than 7% of the athletes met radiographic criteria for splenomegaly, with a baseline splenic length of 13 cm or larger [20]. Because of the wide variability of normal spleen size encountered in these athletes, a specific cut point used to define splenic enlargement seems unreliable. Consequently, obtaining a single sonographic measurement in athletes who have IM needs to be interpreted with caution. For example, an athlete who has IM and a spleen length of 11.5 cm would be considered normal, but this individual might have a baseline of 8 cm, indicating relative splenomegaly. Alternatively, an athlete who has a baseline splenic length of 15 cm could erroneously be labeled as having pathologic splenomegaly [20]. Because of the wide variability of spleen size encountered in this study, the use of imaging techniques to make return-to-play decisions should be used vigilantly, and serial measurements should be considered.

Return-to-play Considerations

The decision of when to return an athlete to activity following acute IM illness is typically very challenging. Because of a lack of scientific evidence available to give clear guidance, return-to-play decisions are often driven by resolution of clinical symptoms.

In most athletes, a period of incapacitation during the height of clinical symptoms should be expected. During this time, it is not usually hard to convince an athlete or a coach that the individual should sit out and rest. It is more difficult, however, to "hold out" an athlete after he or she is feeling well. There is some evidence to suggest that aerobic capacity is not altered and that there are no detrimental effects of light physical activity in individuals who have IM after resolution of fever [21]. Under this premise, when an athlete is asymptomatic, light activity (avoiding any contact and activities involving the Valsalva maneuver) may be permissible. Progression of training may continue based on the individual athlete's clinical response.

Returning an athlete to contact activity is fraught with controversy. When an athlete feels well, the fear of splenic rupture is the most restricting potential complication limiting return to contact activity. It is generally believed that the risk for splenic rupture with IM is greatest in the first 3 weeks of the illness [2].

The rationale behind this theory is that the spleen has achieved maximum enlargement and has begun regressing in size by this time in the course of the illness. Preliminary data from a recent study support this notion. Hosey and colleagues [22] prospectively studied 13 athletes who had acute IM, using ultrasonography to document changes in splenic dimensions. Measurements were compared with existing baseline data obtained during preparticipation examinations. In these athletes, maximum splenic enlargement occurred an average of 10.7 days from the onset of symptoms, and all had reached peak enlargement by 21 days from symptom onset. Although this information lends credence to the notion that the spleen maybe most vulnerable during the initial phase of illness, it does not address risk of rupture. Clinical studies designed to address the risk of splenic rupture at varying degrees of splenic enlargement or at different times of return to activity are not practical or ethical. As such, it is unlikely that there will be concrete objective data on which to base return-to-activity decisions.

Without quality randomized controlled trials to help formulate return-to-play criteria, the use of consensus guidelines that assimilate available evidence is reasonable. The most recent preparticipation physical examination monograph [23] suggested the following guideline for athletes who have IM: a 3-week recovery period, with no physical activity from time of symptom onset, followed by resumption of light activities in asymptomatic individuals in the fourth week, and return to full participation in the fifth week. The use of any guideline should be a starting point for discussion with athletes, coaches, and sports medicine professionals. The most appropriate medical management will likely be achieved by tailoring the treatment plan to the individual athlete and the athlete's specific situation.

MENINGITIS

Meningitis is a potentially life-threatening medical emergency associated with multiple neurologic complications and sequelae. A retrospective analysis, looking at outcomes in adults treated with appropriate antibiotics for pneumococcal meningitis, revealed that only 47% of adults had a good outcome, with 75% of patients having neurologic complications [24]. It is fortunate that most of the reported meningitis cases in the literature concerning athletes are described as aseptic. Multiple case reports have described aseptic meningitis outbreaks among high school football players between 1978 and 1990 [25–30].

Aseptic meningitis refers to cases in which there is clinical and laboratory evidence for meningeal inflammation in the absence of positive bacterial cultures. The primary cause of aseptic meningitis is infection with Enteroviruses (echovirus, coxsackieviruses A and B, polioviruses, and the numbered enteroviruses) [31–33]. "Enteroviruses are responsible for 55% to 70% of all aseptic meningitic cases and for 85% to 95% of cases for which a pathogen is ultimately identified" [33]. Other viral causes include arborviruses, herpesviruses, varicella-zoster virus, adenoviruses, HIV, lymphocytic choriomeningitis virus, measles virus, mumps virus, rubella virus, rabies virus, influenza A and B viruses, parainfluenza virus, parvoviruses, and rotaviruses. There are multiple nonviral causes, many of which are not easily detected by Gram stain and are difficult to culture, often taking weeks to months to grow [33].

Aseptic meningitis is most prevalent during the summer and early fall months (from July to December) [31,32]. Enteroviruses, the primary causative agents, are spread through the fecal-oral route (ie, shared infected water sources, in the form of containers, bottles, or ice cubes). Aseptic meningitis may be more prevalent in fall athletics due to its seasonal predilection and the fecal-oral route of spread [30]. The most common bacterial causes affecting teenagers through 50-year-olds include *Streptococcus pneumoniae* and *Neisseria meningitides*, which make up approximately 80% of all cases. In addition to having an extremely high mortality rate, bacterial meningitis carries an extremely high risk for neurologic sequelae [34].

Aseptic meningitis is a commonly encountered disease process with a clinical presentation similar to that of bacterial meningitis. These similarities can present a diagnostic dilemma. The presentation of meningitis can be acute (<24 hours) or subacute (occurring over 1–7 days) [31,32]. Obvious signs in the clinical presentation of meningitis include the classic triad of fever, headache, and neck stiffness (meningismus) [32,33]. This triad is often accompanied by other nonspecific symptoms including nausea, vomiting, pharyngitis, diarrhea, photophobia, and focal neurologic signs. Symptoms can be accompanied by mental-status changes ranging from lethargy to coma [31–33]. It is important to note that in a clinical series studying bacterial meningitis, only half of the patients over age 16 years presented with the classic triad [31,35]. Clinical presentation may differ based on the age of the affected individual (neonate to elderly). Bacterial meningitis can have a rapidly progressive and fulminant course or an indolent course consisting of vague symptoms. The indolent course is common when an individual has been pretreated with oral antibiotics [32].

History and Physical

There is no substitute for a complete, accurate, and thorough history and physical examination, with particular attention paid to the neurologic examination. The examination may reveal a febrile patient. There may be varying degrees of change in mental status. Focal neurologic signs may be present, which could be associated with a mass versus encephalitis. Papilledema raises concern for a space-occupying lesion versus increased intracranial pressure. Signs of meningeal irritation include meningismus (pain with passive flexion of the neck) and Kernig's and Brudzinski's signs. Kernig's sign is positive if the examiner encounters resistance to passive extension of the knee while the hip is flexed. This test may be done while the patient is supine or seated. Brudzinski's sign occurs when the supine patient has spontaneous flexion of the hips during attempted passive flexion of the neck. Rashes may be characteristic of the offending agent [31,36].

Based on signs/symptoms and physical examination findings, it is virtually impossible to distinguish aseptic from septic bacterial causes of meningitis. Peripheral blood cell counts can be normal or elevated. Cerebrospinal fluid (CSF) analysis is the most important laboratory test for distinguishing aseptic from bacterial meningitis. The CSF fluid should be processed for cell count, protein, glucose, culture, and Gram stain. CSF cultures are positive in 70% to 85% of patients who have not received prior antibiotic therapy but may take up to 48 hours to identify an organism [37].

Imaging

There is debate whether neuroimaging is needed before lumbar puncture (LP) due to the risk of brain herniation in a patient who has elevated intracranial pressure. The true incidence of this complication is unknown and varies based on the study reviewed. The pediatric and adult literature agree that meningitis is a disease process known to result from an inflammatory process associated with increased intracranial pressure. There is inconclusive evidence that herniation occurs secondary to performance of an LP versus as an extension of the inflammatory process. Because of the fear of herniation, there is a growing trend to image all patients before LP. A study involving 301 adults who had bacterial meningitis reported on clinical features at baseline that were associated with abnormal findings on head CT. The study found that patients who had the clinical features noted in (Table 1) were more likely to have abnormal results on CT of the head. Of the 235 patients (78%) who underwent CT before LP, 24% had an abnormal finding but only 5% had mass effect. Of the 96 patients who had none of these abnormalities, only 3 had an abnormal CT scan (1 with mild mass effect). All 3 patients underwent LP without herniation. Among the patients who underwent CT before LP, there was a significant finding of an approximate 2-hour delay in diagnosis and a trend of a 1-hour delay in initiation of admission and administration of empiric antibiotics. Based on these data, the Infectious Disease Society of America (IDSA) made recommendations for which adult patients should undergo CT before LP (see Table 1) [37,38]. The pediatric literature reveals the same concerns involving the increased use of CT before LP, recognizing the potential delay in diagnosis and treatment and the increased risk of radiation exposure in the more radiosensitive pediatric population. Again, the importance of allowing the neurologic examination to define the extent of neurologic abnormalities and to guide decision making for appropriate LP is echoed, with altered mental status, papilledema, and two or more focal neurologic signs being foremost indications

Table 1
The Infectious Disease Society of America recommended criteria for undergoing CT before lumbar puncture in adult patients who have suspected bacterial meningitis

Criteria	Examples
Immunocompromised state	HIV infection or AIDS, immunosuppressive therapy, organ transplantation, chemotherapy
History of central nervous system disease	Mass lesion, stroke, focal infection
New onset seizure	Within 1 week of presentation; some physicians would not perform a lumbar puncture on patients who have prolonged seizures or would delay lumbar puncture for 30 minutes in patients who have short convulsive seizures
Papilledema	Presence of venous pulsations suggests absence of increased intracranial pressure
Abnormal level of consciousness	Can use deteriorating Glascow Coma Score as a tool
Focal neurologic deficit	Dilated nonreactive pupil, abnormalities of ocular motility, abnormal visual fields, gaze palsy, facial palsy, arm or leg drift, abnormal visual fields, abnormal language

Adapted from Tunkel AR, Hartman BJ, Kaplan SL, et al. Practice guidelines for the management of bacterial meningitis. Clin Infect Dis 2004;39:1267–84; and Oliver WJ, Shope TC, Kuhns LR. Fatal lumbar puncture: fact versus fiction—an approach to a clinical dilemma. Pediatrics 2003;112(3):e174–6.

among the pediatric literature [39]. The adult and pediatric literature recognize that CT does not measure intracranial pressure, which has been found to be normal at or about the time of herniation [38,39]. As to whether the previous findings, as discussed in adults or children, should be present on examination, it is suggested that LP be delayed and blood cultures obtained while antibiotics appropriate for age, season, and presenting features are administered. Meanwhile, immediate measures to monitor and reduce intracranial pressure should be initiated, including neurosurgical evaluation along with CT of the head [39]. Approximately 50% to 75% of patients who have bacterial meningitis have positive blood cultures. Meningococcal meningitis has the lowest rate of positive blood cultures [34].

Laboratory Evaluation

Initially, with viral meningitis or encephalitis, CSF samples usually demonstrate a pleocytosis. White cell counts can range from normal to several hundred cells per cubic millimeter [32,33]. Early in the course of the illness, the percentage of polymorphonuclear cells can predominate, but a shift to lymphocytic predominance occurs rapidly [32,33]. A higher white blood cell count is typically encountered in bacterial meningitis. If the Gram stain does not reveal a cause and monocytosis predominates, then viral cultures should be attempted from the original specimen. Polymerase chain reaction (PCR) studies of the CSF can be performed for suspected viral or bacterial causes. PCR examination of CSF is especially valuable when herpes simplex viruses (HSV) or enteroviruses are suspected based on seasonal predilection or history [31–33]. Because of the similarities between CSF findings in aseptic and bacterial meningitis, some clinicians advocate repeat CSF evaluation in stable patients presenting with a subacute presentation, looking for a shift from polymorphonuclear cells to mononuclear cells before antibiotic therapy [31]. CSF glucose should be compared with simultaneous serum glucose. A ratio of 66% is considered normal [31]. In aseptic meningitis, CSF glucose samples are usually within the normal range, with bacterial meningitis causing a drop in CSF glucose [31,33].

Treatment

When neuroimaging is necessary, broad-spectrum, age-appropriate, empiric antibiotics should not be delayed after blood cultures have been obtained [31–33]. See Table 2 for empiric antibiotic treatment for suspected community-acquired bacterial meningitis. More specific antibiotic coverage is added based on results of CSF cultures and the condition of the patient [31,32]. Current treatment guidelines for specific antimicrobial therapy in bacterial meningitis based on isolated pathogen and susceptibility testing are readily available [37]. Adjuvant therapy with early intravenous dexamethasone as an attempt to decrease the rate of neurologic sequelae associated with bacterial meningitis has been evaluated. Animal models have supported the concept of the subarachnoid space inflammatory response being a major factor contributing to mortality and morbidity. Based on a prospective, randomized, placebo-controlled, double-blind multicenter trial by De Gans and colleagues [40], the IDSA has recommended adjunctive intravenous dexamethasone (0.15 mg/kg every 6 hours for 2–4 days) in all adult patients suspected or proven to have pneumococcal meningitis [37]. The De Gans and colleagues' [40] study revealed that mortality was reduced from 15% to 7%, with a relative risk of 0.48 compared with placebo, and that unfavorable outcome was reduced from 25% to 15%, with a relative risk of 0.59 compared with placebo. Significant reductions in mortality (14% versus 34%) and in all unfavorable outcomes (26% versus 52%) were seen only in patients who had *S pneumoniae* meningitis. There was no significant effect of dexamethasone on neurologic sequelae, including hearing loss [37,40]. Dexamethasone should be continued only when the CSF Gram stain reveals gram-positive diplococci or when blood or CSF cultures are positive for

Table 2		
Recommendations for empiric antimicrobial therapy in adolescents and adults who have community-acquired bacterial meningitis		
Age	Common bacterial pathogen	Antibiotic
13–50 y	*Streptococcus pneumoniae, Neisseria meningitidis*	Vancomycin plus a third-generation cephalosporin[a]

[a] Ceftraxone or cefotaxime.

S pneumoniae. The first dose of steroid should be initiated 10 to 20 minutes before or at least in combination with the first dose of antibiotics. Dexamethasone should not be given to an adult patient who has already received antibiotics because this is not been proven to improve patient outcome. At this time, data do not support the use of dexamethasone in adults who have meningitis caused by bacterial pathogens other than *S pneumoniae* [37].

Age-appropriate empiric antibiotics are continued until bacterial causes have been ruled out. Treatment for aseptic meningitis is usually supportive because the course is usually benign. Specific antiviral therapy with acyclovir is indicated for HSV meningitis with encephalitic symptoms [31–33,36]. For unusual nonviral causes of aseptic meningitis (ie, tubercular, spirochetal, rickettsial), specific treatment is indicated [32,33]. Otherwise, the cornerstone of treatment is hydration and antipyretics [31–33,36].

Repeat LP should be considered in patients whose condition has not responded to treatment in 48 hours. Repeat LP is especially important in the care of patients who have penicillin-resistant or cephalosporin-resistant strains of pneumococcal meningitis and who receive adjunctive dexamethasone, which may reduce antimicrobial permeability in the CSF with reduction of inflammation. Gram stain and culture of the CSF should be negative after 24 hours of appropriate antimicrobial therapy [34,37].

Potential Complications

Mortality for bacterial meningitis in the adult population has been reported to be as high as 21%, depending on the causative organism. Pneumococcal meningitis and meningococcal meningitis have mortality rates of 19% to 37% and 3% to 13%, respectively. Upwards of 30% of survivors of pneumococcal meningitis suffer some sort of morbidity, including long-term neurologic sequelae such as hearing loss. Meningococcal meningitis has a morbidity rate of 3% to 7% [34]. The strongest risk factors for poor outcome include patients who have advanced age, indications of systemic compromise, impaired consciousness (low score on Glasgow Coma Scale), low white count in the CSF, positive blood culture, and infection with *S pneumoniae* [34,41]. Focal neurologic deficits are common complications of meningitis and include cranial nerve palsies, monoparesis, hemiparesis, gaze preference, visual field defects, aphasia, ataxia, and impaired cognition [34,41,42]. These neurologic deficits result from a variety of sources including cerebrovascular complications, arterial infarction or vasculitis, venous infarction, hemorrhage, subdural empyema, brain abscess, and myelitis [34]. An eighth cranial nerve deficit resulting in hearing loss is the most frequent cranial nerve abnormality, seen in approximately 14% of meningitis survivors [34,41,42]. Cognitive impairment has been reported to occur in 27% of adults who had good recovery from pneumococcal meningitis. The impairment usually consists of cognitive slowness [34,42].

Prevention

Prevention among athletes revolves around good hand washing and decreasing use of shared water sources. Chemoprophylaxis with antibiotics of persons in close contact with patients who have meningococcal disease is a must for decreasing the risk of contracting the disease. Chemoprophylaxis should be considered in household members, daycare contacts, and anyone directly exposed to the patient's oral secretions and should be administered with in the first few days of the contact's diagnosis. Antibiotics administered after 14 days from onset of disease are probably of limited benefit. Antibiotics that are effective in eliminating risk and nasopharyngeal carriage include rifampin, ciprofloxacin, and ceftriaxone [43]. Special consideration should be given to collegiate athletes who spend a significant amount of time in close contact (eg, dormitories, travel).

Further preventive measures may include the use of individual water bottles and towels, along with proper vaccination. The introduction of effective conjugate vaccination against *Haemophilus influenzae* type b organisms has decreased the incidence of meningitis caused by this organism by more than 99% in countries that have adopted universal immunization [44]. Studies have found that college students residing on campus had at least a three times greater relative risk for contracting meningococcal infection than students living off campus [45]. The incidence of meningococcal disease for college freshman living in dormitories reaches 5.1 per 100,000 compared with all undergraduates combined, at a rate of 0.7 per 100,000 [46]. It is believed that approximately 70% to 80% of serogroups that cause meningococcal disease in adolescents and young adults are possibly preventable by use of the tetravalent conjugate vaccines. Menactra (MCV4) is a tetravalent meningococcal conjugate vaccine containing polysaccharide serogroups to A, C, Y, and W-135 attached to a diphtheria toxoid (protein) that prompts T-cell and B-cell response and provides protective antibodies within 7 to 10 days after vaccination [47]. MCV4 is recommended for administration by the United States Advisory Committee on Immunization practices (ACIP) of the Centers for Disease Control and Prevention (CDC) and the American Academy of Pediatrics as the primary vaccination against meningococcus in the 11- to 55-year age group [47,48].

Return to Play

Return-to-play considerations for athletes who have aseptic meningitis mainly depend on resolution of systemic symptoms including fever, meningismus, and headache. There is a lack of evidence on which to base return-to-play decisions for athletes recovering from viral meningitis. In general, a convalescent period of symptom recovery should be expected to last several days to weeks. A gradual return to activity, slowly increasing in intensity after clinical symptoms have resolved, should be anticipated. Return to competition following recovery from bacterial meningitis depends more on the presence of secondary sequelae and comorbidities. All patients who survive bacterial meningitis require formal hearing evaluations [49]. These patients would also benefit from formal neuropsychologic evaluation, especially if infected with *S pneumoniae*, to evaluate cognition, memory, attention and executive functioning, and reaction speed. Most abnormalities are identified in the areas of visuospatial reasoning, speed in performing attention and executive functioning tests, and reaction speed [50]. Survivors of bacterial meningitis who have limb amputation, end organ damage, and neurologic sequelae require long-term multidisciplinary rehabilitation [49].

SEXUALLY TRANSMITTED DISEASES

This section highlights a growing problem seen in the adolescent and young adult population in the United States and discusses recommendations for screening, diagnostic tests, and guidelines for participation in athletes infected with common STDs. The training room offers an environment that is safe and convenient to the athlete, often providing athletes their only form of medical care. The training room is often the setting in which concerns about potential STDs or exposure to STDs are revealed to the sports medicine specialist. Comprehensive guidelines for diagnosing and treating STDs can be found in the 2002 CDC report, "Sexually Transmitted Diseases Treatment Guidelines" [51].

A multicenter, cross-sectional study looking at lifestyle and health risks of collegiate athletes found that college athletes appear to be at higher risk than their nonathletic peers for certain maladaptive lifestyle behaviors including less-safe sex, greater number of sexual partners, and less contraceptive use [52]. Perhaps these behaviors, in part, have contributed to an increased prevalence of STDs seen in adolescents and young adults. Recent research has indicated a high prevalence of asymptomatic *Chlamydia* infection in young adults aged 18 to 26 years. This increased prevalence reveals significant racial and ethnic disparities in chlamydial and gonococcal infections [53]. The highest rates of *Chlamydia* infection have been reported in the 15- to 24-year age group. HIV infection is the second leading cause of morbidity in the world and is contracted most commonly by individuals aged 15 to 25 years. Human papillomavirus (HPV) is the most widespread STD in the world. The CDC estimates that 50% to 75% of sexually active men and women acquire HPV at some point in their lives. It has also been estimated that 35% of teens and young adults in various Western countries have acquired HPV. Approximately 20% of the United States adult population is infected with HSV, which represents a 30% increase over the last 25 years [54]. The staggering reality associated with these statistics is that they belong to the very population that sports medicine specialists spend most of their time treating: adolescents and young adults.

In the 2002 CDC report, the major strategies for the prevention and control of STDs are outlined. These strategies revolve around education and counseling about safer sexual behaviors in persons at risk; identification of asymptomatic persons and symptomatic persons unlikely to seek diagnostic and treatment services; effective diagnosis and treatment; evaluation, treatment, and counseling of sexual partners of persons who have STDs; and pre-exposure immunizations for vaccine-preventable STDs in selected populations [51,55].

Sports medicine physicians provide a key role in the identification of individuals who could be afflicted with STDs. These physicians are often the only contact these individuals have with a health care professional during their college years, providing an excellent format for identification, treatment, and counseling/education of infected individuals.

Screening Practices

The CDC recommends the screening of all sexually active women younger than 24 years of age whether symptomatic or asymptomatic. Women older than 24 years of age should be screened if they are at risk for chlamydial infection (ie, new sexual partner or history of multiple partners) [51,55]. With the high national prevalence of *Chlamydia* infection (4% of all young adults) and gonorrheal infection (in minorities), screening strategies appear to be failing [53]. This failure could be due to such screening inadequacies as (1) the lack of CDC recommendations for screening young males (who represent a significant reservoir for asymptomatic *Chlamydia* infection); (2) the evidence that CDC screening recommendations for young women are not widely observed; and (3) the lack of connection between young adults and health care professionals [53,56]. Screening in the young adult population makes sense. Studies looking at screening for STDs during preparticipation sports examination found the prevalence of chlamydial and gonococcal infections in young women to be 6.5% and 2.0%, respectively; in young men, the prevalence was 2.8% and 0.7%, respectively. Of the individuals who were infected, 93.1% had no symptoms [57]. Studies in adolescents have documented short periods (4.7–7.6 months) until re-infection occurs, suggesting that sexually active adolescents should be screened every 6 months [56]. Studies have revealed that it is more cost-effective to screen all high-risk women (based on age, high-risk behavior, or both) than to screen symptomatic women only, based on decreasing downstream health care dollars [56]. Testing for HIV should be offered to all individuals who seek evaluation for STDs or who are diagnosed with syphilis. Complete recommendations for STD testing can be found in the CDC 2002 report [51].

Urethritis/Cervicitis

The principal bacterial pathogens causing urethritis and cervicitis are *N gonorrhoeae* and *C trachomatis* [51,55]. Urethritis and cervicitis are easily identified by urethral or cervical discharge of mucopurulent or purulent material. Symptoms in men, however, may be as vague as dysuria or urethral puritis. Common symptoms in women include odorless vaginal discharge, vaginal bleeding (usually after intercourse), and dysparenunia. Many women, however, remain asymptomatic [55]. When infection of the endocervix ascends in women, pelvic inflammatory infection can develop, resulting in systemic symptoms of fever and abdominal pain. When infection ascends in men, it can result in epididymitis or epididymo-orchitis with unilateral testicular pain and may present without discharge or dysuria [51,55,58,59]. Epididymtitis and epididymo-orchitis are the most common causes of acute scrotum in adolescent boys and young men and must be distinguished from testicular torsion with prompt examination and ultrasound [58,59].

Between 10% and 30% of patients who have a gonorrheal infection have a concomitant chlamydial infection. For this reason, tests for *N gonorrhoeae* and *Chlamydia* are performed at the same time. Laboratory diagnosis of urogenital disease in women should include endocervical culture or nucleic amplification testing for *N gonorrhoeae* and *C trachomatis*. *Ureaplasma urealyticum* and *Mycoplasma genitalium* should be considered in men who have urethritis if *N gonorrhoeae* and *Chlamydia* are determined to not be causative factors [51].

The CDC recommends a low threshold for diagnosing pelvic inflammatory disease (PID) because of the significant associated sequelae, including infertility. Empiric treatment is recommended for suspected PID in women at risk for STDs who have uterine, adnexal, or cervical motion tenderness. Other associated criteria for PID include abnormal vaginal or cervical mucopurulent discharge, elevated C-reactive protein level or erythrocyte sedimentation rate, history of chlamydial and gonococcal infections, oral temperature greater than 101°F (38.3°C), or white blood cells present on saline preparation of vaginal secretions.

Disseminated gonococcal infection including septic emboli (resulting in polyarticular tenosynovitis and dermatitis) and septic arthritis can occur in 1% to 3% of adults who have gonorrhea. The joints commonly involved include those of the wrists, ankles, hands, and feet. The axial skeleton is rarely involved. Initial aspiration of the joint may be negative for infection, but untreated disease results in septic arthritis, usually involving the elbows, wrists, knees, or ankles [51,55].

Treatment options for the infections discussed in the previous text are well established and accessible through the CDC [51]. Hospitalization is warranted for patients who have PID and epididymitis with or without orchitis when the patient is deemed unreliable to complete treatment, as can be the case with adolescents. There is no efficacy comparing parenteral with oral regimens in PID or epididymitis/epididymo-orchitis. Usually, there is substantial improvement within 3 days after initiation of treatment. Failure to respond should prompt the clinician to consider alternative diagnoses or extension of disease. Hospitalization and parenteral therapy is required for initial therapy for disseminated gonococcal infection, and transitioning to an appropriate oral regimen is dictated by patient improvement and clinical judgment. In instances of septic arthritis, consultation with an orthopedic specialist is required to allow proper decontamination of the joint space [51].

Follow-up is required when the athlete remains symptomatic despite adequate treatment. Symptoms alone, without documentation of laboratory evidence of infection, are not a sufficient basis for re-treatment. Patients who have simple urethritis, cervicitis, or rectal disease should refrain from sexual intercourse until 7 days after therapy is started. Re-treatment may be warranted if symptoms persist, if there is a history of noncompliance with initial treatment, or if the patient was re-exposed to an untreated sex partner (the usual cause for infection after adequate treatment). Otherwise, a culture of an intraurethral swab specimen for *Trichomonas vaginalis* should be obtained. Some cases of continued or recurrent urethritis may be secondary to tetracycline-resistant *U urealyticum*. If a patient is treated with doxycycline or azithromycin for *Chlamydia* infection, test of cure is not recommended. Test of cure is recommended 3 weeks after completion of erythromycin therapy for *Chlamydia* infection. Test of cure should not be performed until 3 weeks after completion of therapy because of high false positive results [51]. Due to the high rate of re-infection with *Chlamydia* in adolescent and young women, many experts recommend screening at 3 to 4 months following treatment [51,56].

Return to play
Return-to-play decisions are made based on the disease process. Simple/uncomplicated urethritis/cervicitis/rectal disease does not require much if any time away from practice and competition. In athletes affected with PID, epididymitis, epididymo-orchitis, or disseminated gonorrheal disease, systemic improvement dictates return to sport, including resolution of fever, pain, nausea, and vomiting. If infection includes the diagnosis of a septic joint, more time is required for recovery and physical therapy for decontamination of the invasion of the joint space. Recovery time depends on whether arthroscopy or an open procedure was performed and on any sequelae related to joint mobility (ie, scarring/arthrofibrosis).

Diseases Characterized by Vaginal Discharge
Bacterial vaginosis
Bacterial vaginosis occurs secondary to the replacement of normal vaginal flora (*Lactobacillus* sp) with anaerobic microorganisms (ie, *Prevotella* sp and *Mobiluncus* sp), *Gardnerella vaginalis*, and *Mycoplasma hominis*. It is the most common cause of vaginal discharge. Most women are asymptomatic, but symptoms can include vaginal discharge, vulvar itching or irritation, and vaginal odor [51,55]. Bacterial vaginosis is associated with having multiple sex partners, douching, and lack of vaginal lactobacilli. It is unclear whether it is a sexually transmitted infection. Diagnosis is based on Gram stain or clinical criteria including a homogenous, white, noninflammatory discharge that smoothly coats the vaginal walls; the presence of clue cells on microscopic examination; a vaginal fluid pH of greater than 4.5; and a fishy odor before or after addition of 10% potassium hydroxide (positive whiff test). Symptomatic disease in all women and asymptomatic disease in high-risk pregnant women must be treated based on the strategies outlined by the CDC [51].

Trichomoniasis
Trichomoniasis is caused by the protozoan *Trichomonas vaginalis*. Most men do not have symptoms. Women have symptoms characterized by diffuse, malodorous, yellow-green discharge with vulvar irritation, although some women are asymptomatic. The easiest form of diagnosis is based on visualization of

trichomonads by microscopy of vaginal secretions. Culture offers the most sensitive method of diagnosis. Numerous antitrichomonal treatment options are available and effective [51,55].

Human Papillomavirus Infection

There are more than 30 types of HPV that are species specific and infect the human genital tract [51,60]. Most infections are asymptomatic, unrecognized, or subclinical, leading to a high transmission rate. Infectivity does not correlate to the presence or absence of visible lesions. Transmission can occur by direct skin-to-skin contact. Incubation can range from weeks to years depending on the immune status of the patient [61]. The most apparent manifestation of genital HPV is genital warts (condylomata acuminata), which are caused by HPV types 6 and 11 [51,60]. These warts can present as single or multiple papules on the penis, scrotum, vulva, cervix, vagina, perineum, anal region, urethra, and mouth. Lesions generally appear as flesh colored to gray, hyperkeratotic, exophytic, and sessile or pedunculated.

Untreated warts can resolve spontaneously, remain unchanged, or increase in size or number. Treatment options are dictated by the preference of the patient and the experience of the health care provider. Wart number, size, morphology, and anatomic site may influence the type of treatment provided. Many patients require a course of treatments rather than a single treatment. Patient-applied therapies and provider-administered therapies are available [51,60].

Prevention incorporates the use of routine Papanicolaou smear (Pap smear) screening and vaccination. The Pap smear is a successful screening tool for detecting cervical dysplasia, which can be a subclinical presentation for HPV infection. With each Pap smear, a high-risk HPV-DNA panel is performed to detect high-risk HPV types 16, 18, 31, 33, 35, 39, 45, 51, 52, 56, 58, 59, and 68 in conjunction with cervical cytology. This panel for detection of high-risk HPV types is associated with a high sensitivity of 98% and a high negative predictive value of 99%. The HPV-DNA screen allows identification of women who have the disease and those who are at risk of developing the disease in the future. Further treatment is dictated by the risk of HPV type and the cytology results from the Pap smear [60]. Vaccinating against HPV is based on preventing the second most common malignant disease in women by immunizing against the two most common oncogenic types, HPV-16 and HPV-18, which are associated with 50% and 20% of cervical cancer, respectively [61]. By adding immunization against low-risk HPV genotypes 6 and 11, another 12% of low-grade cervical lesions and most cases of genital warts can be prevented [62]. In 2005, a randomized, double-blind, placebo-controlled trial assessed the efficacy of a three-dose vaccine in 552 women aged 16 to 23 years and revealed that a combined incidence of persistent infection or disease with HPV 6, 11, 16, or 18 fell by 90% compared with placebo. The vaccine appears to be safe and well tolerated [63]. Based on these and similar study results, the Food and Drug Administration approved licensure of the first cervical cancer vaccine in the United States on June 8, 2006. This quadrivalent HPV (types 6, 11, 16, and 18) recombinant vaccine prevents cervical cancer and cervical, vulvar, and vaginal lesions caused by HPV types 6, 11, 16, and 18 and is licensed for use in 9- to 26-year-old girls and women as a three-dose series. The target for routine immunization is 11- to 12-year-olds [64]. Clinical trials are underway for evaluating the efficacy of vaccinating men [65].

Return to play

There are no specific rules for return to play in athletes who have condylomata acuminata. If condylomata acuminata occur in the oral region, it is advisable to base decisions for play on the 2004 recommendations of the National Collegiate Athletics Association (NCAA) regarding wrestlers who have molluscum contagiosum. Because of the contagious nature of these lesions, it is recommended to cover solitary and clustered lesions with a gas-permeable membrane such as Op-Site (Smith and Nephew plc., London, United Kingdom), followed by wrap and stretch tape. If the lesions cannot be adequately covered, then play must be restricted until adequate treatment is obtained [66,67].

Genital Ulcer Disease

Genital herpes

Genital herpes is a recurrent, life-long viral infection caused by two serotypes, HSV-1 (30% of cases) and HSV-2 (70% of cases) [51]. Both serotypes can be present in oral and genital secretions [55]. Most persons infected with HSV-2 infections have not been diagnosed, which allows unrecognized shedding of the virus in the genital track with transmission by persons unaware of their infection [51]. Infection is divided into primary infection, in which patients do not have antibodies to HSV-1 or HSV-2; recurrent infection, caused by reactivation of genital HSV; and asymptomatic infection, characterized by viral shedding (could be responsible for up to 70% of transmission and latent infection) [51,55,68].

The physical presentation is highly variable and nonspecific. Initial presentation can be marked by painful genital ulcers, dysuria, tender local lymphadenopathy, and systemic symptoms such as fever, headache, and malaise. Outbreaks can be preceded by prodromal symptoms consisting of local tingling/burning and discomfort. Primary eruptions are usually complicated by more systemic symptoms, whereas recurrent eruptions are usually milder in relation to lesion outbreak and rarely have systemic symptoms. Primary lesions last between 2 and 6 weeks and can be extremely painful. Viral shedding can last approximately 15 to 16 days, with new lesions forming for about 10 days following infection. Women tend to suffer from more severe disease. In recurrent outbreaks, symptoms are milder, with fewer lesions and viral shedding lasting about 3 days [69]. Diagnosis is made by viral culture. Sensitivity decreases the longer the ulcer/lesions are present. PCR is highly sensitive but usually reserved for diagnosing herpes meningitis/encephalitis because of its high cost. Distinction of serogroup is important because it influences prognosis and counseling. HSV antibodies form during the first weeks following infection and remain indefinitely, therefore forming the basis of serologic testing and serotyping [51,69]. Treatment includes the use of effective oral antivirals. These medications can be used for initial outbreaks, recurrent outbreaks, and suppressive therapy. Intravenous therapy is reserved for severe or disseminated disease [51,69].

Return to play. In the case of a primary infection, return to activity can be initiated when systemic symptoms have resolved. Depending on the severity of the primary outbreak, resolution of mucous membrane and skin eruptions can take from 2 to 6 weeks. As the outbreak improves, pain should improve concordantly. Nonsteroidal anti-inflammatory drugs (NSAIDs), acetaminophen, or narcotic pain medication may be required. Recurrent outbreaks usually resolve in 8 days and are associated with less pain compared with primary outbreaks and should respond to NSAIDs and acetaminophen [69]. Outbreaks in athletes and teams have been reported in the literature. Transmission occurs from an infected individual to a susceptible host by skin-to-skin contact, especially if the skin barrier is disrupted, resulting in herpes gladiatorum [70,71]. Most discussions regarding return-to-play decisions have focused on the sport of wrestling. The NCAA has published specific guidelines to address this issue. The NCAA recommendations regarding primary infection [66] are summarized as follows:

> The wrestler must be free of systemic symptoms of viral infection, must have developed no new blisters for 72 hours before examination, and must have no moist lesions. All lesions must be dried and surmounted by a firm, adherent crust. The wrester must have been on an appropriate dosage of systemic antiviral therapy for at least 120 hours before and at the time of the meet or tournament, and active herpetic infections shall not be covered to allow participation.

Recurrent infections are similarly dealt with, requiring lesions be healed and appropriate antiviral therapy initiated for a period of at least 120 hours. Wrestlers who have a history of recurrent herpes labialis or herpes gladiatorum should be considered for season-long prophylaxis with appropriate antiviral medication [66,67].

Syphilis

Primary syphilis is usually associated with a single, painless chancre, although multiple chancres can be present and the lesions can be painful on presentation. The chancre is most commonly found on the external genitalia and develops about 10 to 90 days (average, 21 days) after infection and spontaneously resolves in 1 to 4 months [72].

Suspected diagnosis is confirmed on dark-field microscopy of the lesion or by serologic testing. Nontreponemal testing can produce false positive testing due to pregnancy, autoimmune disorders, and infections. False negative results can occur if the sample is not diluted properly, which allows for large amounts of antibody to block the antibody-antigen reaction [51,72]. After adequate treatment, the patient should convert to a nonreactive state; however, some patients maintain a persistent low-level positive treponemal test, referred to as a serofast reaction. Treponemal-specific tests detect antibodies to an antigenic component of *Treponema pallidum*. These tests include the enzyme immunoassay test for antitreponemal IgG, the *Treponema pallidum* hemagglutination test, the microhemagglutination test with *Treponema pallidum* antigen, the fluorescent treponemal antibody-absorption test, and the enzyme-linked immunosorbent assay and are reserved to confirm diagnosis in patients who have a reactive nontreponemal test. Treponemal tests remain positive for life despite treatment, making treponemal-specific titers not useful for assessing treatment efficacy [72].

Treatment of primary syphilis is based on test results and clinical suspicion (if a test result is believed to be a false negative). Patients can develop a reaction known as the Jarisch-Herxheimer reaction within 24 hours of treatment, which results in an acute febrile reaction frequently accompanied by headache, myalgias, and other constitutional symptoms, and is most commonly seen with treatment for early syphilis. Antipyretics can be used but have not been proven to prevent this reaction [51,72]. At 6 to 12 months, the patient should be re-examined and should undergo repeat serologic testing to confirm successful treatment. Treatment failure consists of recurrent symptoms or a sustained fourfold increase in nontreponemal test titers despite appropriate treatment. Treatment failure may lead to the development of secondary or tertiary syphilis.

Secondary syphilis develops weeks to months after the initial chancre appears. At this stage, the skin is most often affected with macular, maculopapular, or pustular lesions that begin on the trunk and proximal extremities including the palms of the hands and soles of the feet. Condyloma latum is a soft, verucous plaque usually found in warm, moist areas such as the perineum and perianal skin. This eruption is painless but highly infectious. The renal, liver, central nervous system, and musculoskeletal system can also be affected. The diagnosis is confirmed by nontreponemal and treponemal-specific tests. Treatment and follow-up is the same as for primary syphilis [72].

Tertiary syphilis is classified into gummatous, cardiovascular, and neurosyphilis. Gummatous syphilis consists of gummas, which are granulomatous-like lesions that can cause local destruction of tissue—namely, skin, mucous membranes, and bone. Any organ system, however, can be affected. Cardiac involvement can present as aortitis with the formation of aneurysms or the destruction of elastic tissue in the aorta. Neurosyphilis (manifesting as seizures, ataxia, aphasia, paresis, hyper-reflexia, personality or cognitive changes, visual changes, hearing loss, neuropathy, and loss of bowel or bladder function) can affect up to 10% of people who have untreated syphilis.

Current treatment recommendations are available from the CDC [51].

Return to play. Due to the highly contagious nature of these lesions, return to play should be restricted in athletes who have skin lesions until adequate treatment is completed and there is resolution of the lesions. If the athlete is affected by tertiary syphilis, then return to play is dictated by resolution of systemic symptoms and related sequelae.

Chancroid

Chancroid is a cofactor for HIV transmission and is often (10% of persons) associated with *Treponema pallidum* or HSV in coinfection. If chancroid is suspected, diagnosis requires identification of *Haemophilus ducreyi* on special culture media (sensitivity ≤80%). Diagnosis should be considered when the following criteria are met:

1. The patient has one or more painful ulcers.
2. The patient has no evidence of *Treponema pallidum* infection by dark-field microscopy examination of ulcer exudate or by a serologic test for syphilis performed at least 7 days after onset of ulcers.
3. A test for HSV performed on the ulcer exudate is negative.

The typical clinical presentation for chancroid occurs in one third of patients and consists of a combination of painful ulcers and tender inguinal lymphadenopathy. When accompanied by suppurative inguinal adenopathy, these findings are almost pathognomonic for chancroid [51].

Return to play. Appropriate antibiotic administration typically results in the resolution of clinical symptoms and prevents transmission to other people [51]. Return to play can commence with adequate pain control and resolution of suppurative lesions.

In light of the increased prevalence of STDs, it is important for health care providers to provide greater emphasis on prevention and management of STDs. This is especially true for sports medicine specialists, in light of their primary patient population. The goal should be to promote a program that is comprehensive in its screening, recognition, and management of STDs, including the recognition and education of athletes practicing high-risk behaviors.

SUMMARY

Collegiate athletes are exposed to a host of infectious diseases. Most resultant illnesses are mild and self-limited. Potential complications involving significant morbidity and even mortality, although uncommon, do occur. Sports medicine practitioners are often the first line of defense against infectious diseases. In dealing with collegiate athletes, an in-depth knowledge of commonly encountered infectious diseases is paramount to the recognition, management, and development of prevention strategies.

References

[1] Papesch M, Watkins R. Epstein-Barr virus infectious mononucleosis. Clin Otolaryngol 2001;26(1):3–8.
[2] Maki DG, Reich RM. Infectious mononucleosis in the athlete. Diagnosis, complications, and management. Am J Sports Med 1982;10(3):162–73.
[3] MacKnight JM. Infectious mononucleosis: ensuring a safe return to sport. Phys Sportsmed 2002;30(1):27–8.

[4] Hoagland RJ. Infectious mononucleosis. Prim Care 1975;2:295–307.

[5] Sevier TL. Infectious disease in athletes. Med Clin of North Am 1994;78(2):389–412.

[6] Farley DR, Zietlow SP, Bannon MP, et al. Spontaneous rupture of the spleen due to infectious mononucleosis. Mayo Clin Proc 1992;67:846–53.

[7] Frelinger DP. The ruptured spleen in college athletes: a preliminary report. J Am Coll Health Assoc 1978;26:217.

[8] Johnson MA, Cooperberg PL, Boisvert J, et al. Spontaneous splenic rupture in infectious mononucleosis. AJR Am J Roentgenol 1981;136:11–114.

[9] Tamayo SG, Rickman LS, Mathews WC, et al. Examiner dependence on physical diagnostic tests for the detection of splenomegaly: a prospective study with multiple observers. J Gen Intern Med 1993;8(2):69–75.

[10] Ayers AB. The spleen. In: Grainger RG, Allison DJ, editors. Diagnostic radiology: an anglo-american textbook of imaging. 2nd edition. Edinburgh (UK): Churchill Livingstone; 1992. p. 2403.

[11] Fried AM. Retroperitoneum, pancreas, spleen, and lymph nodes. In: McGahan JP, Goldberg BB, editors. Diagnostic ultrasound: a logical approach. Philadelphia: Lippincott–Raven Publishers; 1998. p. 777.

[12] Meire H, Farrant P. The liver. In: Baxter GM, Allan PLP, Morley P, editors. Clinical diagnostic ultrasound. Oxford (UK): Blackwell Science Ltd; 1999. p. 379–80.

[13] Loftus WK, Metrewili C. Normal splenic size in a Chinese population. J Ultrasound Med 1997;16:345–7.

[14] Konus O. Normal liver, spleen, and kidney dimensions in neonates, infants, and children: evaluation with sonography. AJR Am J Roentgenol 1998;171:1693–8.

[15] Megremis SD, Vlachonikolis IG, Tsilimigaki AM. Spleen length in childhood with US: normal values based on age, sex, and somatometric parameters. Radiology 2004;231:129–34.

[16] Rosenberg HK, Markowitz RI, Kolberg H, et al. Normal splenic size in infants and children: sonographic measurements. AJR Am J Roentgenol 1991;157:119–21.

[17] Loftus WK, Chow LT, Metreweli C. Sonographic measurement of splenic length: correlation with measurement at autopsy. J Clin Ultrasound 1999;27:71–4.

[18] Capaccioli L, Stecco A, Vanzi E, et al. Ultrasonographic study on the growth and dimensions of healthy children and adult organs. Intal J Anat Embryol 2000;105(1):1–50.

[19] DeLand FH. Normal spleen size. Radiology 1970;97:589–92.

[20] Hosey RG, Mattacola CG, Kriss V, et al. Ultrasound assessment of spleen size in collegiate athletes. Br J Sports Med 2006;40(3):251–4.

[21] Welch MJ, Wheeler L. Aerobic capacity after contracting infectious mononucleosis. J Orthop Sports Phys Ther 1986;8:199–202.

[22] Hosey RG, Jagger J, Kriss V, et al. Ultrasonographic evaluation of splenomegaly in athletes with acute infectious mononucleosis. Presented at the 15th annual meeting of the American Medical Society for Sports Medicine. Miami (FL), April 2006.

[23] Matheson GO, Boyajian-O'Neill LA, Cardone D, et al. Preparticipation physical evaluation monograph. Wappes JR, editor. 3rd edition. Minneapolis (MN): McGraw Hill; 2004. p. 1–98.

[24] Kastenbauer S, Pfister HW. Pneumococcal meningitis in adults, spectrum of complications and prognostic factors in a series of 87 cases. Brain 2003;126:1015–25.

[25] Moore M, Baron RC, Filstein MR, et al. Aseptic meningitis and high school football players, 1978 and 1980. JAMA 1983;249(15):2039–42.

[26] Centers for Disease Control. Aseptic meningitis in a high school football team, Ohio. MMWR Morb Mortal Wkly Rep 1981;29:631–7.

[27] Baron RC, Hatch MH, Kleeman K, et al. Aseptic meningitis among members of a high school football team. JAMA 1982;248(14):1724–7.

[28] Thomas JC. Aseptic meningitis in football players. J Sch Health 1990;60(1):11.

[29] Alexander JP, Chapman LE, Pallansch MA, et al. Coxsackeivirus B$_2$ infection and aseptic meningitis; a focal outbreak among members of a high school football team. J Infect Dis 1993;167:1201–5.

[30] Goodman RA, Thacker SB, Solomon SL, et al. Infectious diseases in competitive sports. JAMA 1994;16(11):862–7.

[31] Moeller JL. Aseptic meningitis: a seasonal concern. Physician and Sportsmedicine 1997;25(7):34–42.

[32] Rajnik M, Ottolini MG. Serious infections of the central nervous system: encephalitis, meningitis, and brain abscess. Adolesc Med 2000;11(2):401–24.

[33] Coyle PK. Overview of acute and chronic meningitis. Neurol Clin 1999;17(4):691–709.

[34] Van de Beek D, de Grans J, Tunkel AR, et al. Community-acquired bacterial meningitis in adults. N Engl J Med 2006;354(1):44–53.

[35] Sigurdardottir B, Bjornsson OM, Jonsdottir KE, et al. Diagnosis of bacterial meningitis in adults: a 20 year review. Arch Intern Med 1997;151:425–30.

[36] Nelson S, Sealy DP. The aseptic meningitis syndrome. Am Fam Physician 1993;48(5):809–15.

[37] Tunkel AR, Hartman BJ, Kaplan SL, et al. Practice guidelines for the management of bacterial meningitis. Clin Infect Dis 2004;39:1267–84.

[38] Hasbun R, Abrahams J, Jekel J, et al. Computed tomography of the head before lumbar puncture in adults with suspected meningitis. N Engl J Med 2001;345(24):1727–33.

[39] Oliver WJ, Shope TC, Kuhns LR. Fatal lumbar puncture: fact versus fiction—an approach to a clinical dilemma. Pediatrics 2003;112(3):e174–6.

[40] de Gans J, van de Beek D. Dexamethasone in adults with bacterial meningitis. N Engl J Med 2002;347(20):1549–56.

[41] Van de Beek D, Gans Jd, Spanjaard L, et al. Clinical features and prognostic factors in adults with bacterial meningitis. N Engl J Med 2004;351(18):1849–59.

[42] Aronin SI, Peduzzi P, Quagliarello VJ, et al. Community-acquired bacterial meningitis: risk stratification for adverse clinical outcome and effect of antibiotic timing. Ann Intern Med 1998;129(11):862–9.

[43] Rosentein NE, Perkins BA, Stephens DS, et al. Meningococcal disease. N Engl J Med 2006;344(18):1378–88.

[44] Saez-Llorens X, McCracken GH. Bacterial meningitis in children. Lancet 2003;361:2139–48.

[45] Harrison LH, Dwyer DM, Maples CT, et al. Risk of meningococcal infection in college students. JAMA 1999;281:1906–10. Published correction appears in JAMA 2000;283:2659.

[46] Bruce MG, Rosentein NE, Capparella JM, et al. Risk factors for meningococcal disease in college students. JAMA 2001;286:688–93.

[47] Kimel SR. Prevention of meningococcal disease. Am Fam Physician 2005;72:2049–56.

[48] American Academy of Pediatrics Policy Statement from Committee on Infectious Diseases. Prevention and control of meningococcal disease: recommendations for use of meningococcal vaccines in pediatric patients. Pediatrics 2005;116:496–505.

[49] Welch SB, Nadel S. Treatment of meningococcal infection. Arch Dis Child 2003;88:608–14.

[50] Van de Beek D, Schmand B, de Gans J, et al. Cognitive impairment in adults with good recovery after bacterial meningitis. J Infect Dis 2002;186:1047–52.

[51] Centers for Disease Control and Prevention. Sexually transmitted diseases treatment guidelines. MMWR Morb Mortal Weekly Rep 2002;51(RR-6):1–78.

[52] Nattiv A, Puffer JC, Green GA. Lifestyles and health risks of collegiate athletes: a multi-center study. Clin J Sport Med 1997;7:262–72.

[53] Miller WC, Ford CA, Morris M, et al. Prevalence of chlamydial and gonococcal infections among young adults in the United States. JAMA 2004;291(18):2229–36.

[54] Genuis SJ, Genuis SK. Managing the sexually transmitted disease pandemic: a time for reevaluation. Am J Obstet Gynecol 2004;191(4):1103–12.

[55] Miller KE, Ruiz DE, Graves JC. Update on the prevention and treatment of sexually transmitted diseases. Am Fam Physician 2003;67(9):379–86.

[56] Spigarelli MG, Biro FM. Sexually transmitted disease testing: evaluation of diagnostic tests and methods. Adolesc Med 2004;15:287–99.

[57] Nsuami M, Elie M, Brooks BN, et al. Screening for sexually transmitted diseases during pre-participation sports examination of high school adolescents. J Adolesc Health 2003;32(5): 336–9.

[58] O'Brien WM, Lynch JH. The acute scrotum. Am Fam Physician 1988;37(3):239–47.

[59] Dogra V, Bhatt S. Acute painful scrotum. Radiol Clin North Am 2004;42:349–63.

[60] Krejici EB, Sanchez ML. Genital human papillomavirus infection. Clinics In Family Practice 2005;7(1):79–96.

[61] Munoz N. Against which human papillomavirus types shall we vaccinate and screen? The international perspective. Int J Cancer 2004;111:278.

[62] ALTS Group. Human papillomavirus testing for triage of women with cytologic evidence of low-grade sqaumous intraepithelial lesions: baseline data from a randomized trial: the Atypical Squamous Cells of Undetermined Significance/Low-Grade Sqaumous Intraepithelial Lesions Triage Study (ALTS) Group. J Natl Cancer Inst 2000;107:397–402.

[63] Villa LL, Costa RL, Petta CA, et al. Prophylactic quadrivalent human papillomavirus (types 6, 11, 16, and 18) L1 virus-like particle vaccine in young women: a randomized double-blind placebo-controlled multicentre phase II efficacy trial. Lancet Oncol 2005;6:271–8.

[64] FDA approves licensure of first U.S. HPV vaccine. American Academy Pediatrics News 2006;27(7):5.

[65] DeNoon D. Cervical cancer vaccine approved: FDA approves Gardasil for girls and women aged 9–26. Available at: http://www.webmd.com/content/Article/123/115099.htm. Accessed June, 2006.

[66] Bubb RS-RE, NCAA Wrestling Committee. 2004 NCAA Wrestling rules and interpretations. In: Bubb RG, editor. NCAA guideline 2b. Indianapolis (IN): The National Collegiate Athletic Association; 2004.

[67] Cordoro KM, Ganz JE. Training room management of medical conditions: sports dermatology. Clin Sports Med 2005;24:565–98.

[68] Mertz GJ, Benedetti J, Ashley R, et al. Risk factors for the sexual transmission of genital herpes. Ann Intern Med 1992;116:197.

[69] Beauman JG. Genital herpes: a review. Am Fam Physician 2005;72:1527–34.

[70] Becker TM, Kodsi R, Bailey P, et al. Grappling with herpes: herpes gladiatorum. Am J Sports Med 1988;166(6):665–9.

[71] Belongia EA, Goodman JL, Holland EJ, et al. An outbreak of herpes gladiatorum at a high-school wrestling camp. N Engl J Med 1991;325(13):906–10.

[72] Brown DL, Frank JE. Diagnosis and management of syphilis. Am Fam Physician 2003;68: 283–90.

Clin Sports Med 26 (2007) 473–487

CLINICS IN SPORTS MEDICINE

ELSEVIER
SAUNDERS

Infectious Disease and the Extreme Sport Athlete

Craig C. Young, MD[a,b,*], Mark W. Niedfeldt, MD[a,b,c],
Laura M. Gottschlich, DO[b], Charles S. Peterson, MD[d],
Matthew R. Gammons, MD[b,e]

[a]Department of Orthopaedic Surgery, Medical College of Wisconsin, 9200 W.
Wisconsin Ave., Milwaukee, WI 53226, USA
[b]Department of Family and Community Medicine, Medical College of Wisconsin,
9200 W. Wisconsin Ave., Milwaukee, WI 53226, USA
[c]Department of Cell Biology, Neurobiology, and Anatomy, Medical College of Wisconsin,
9200 W. Wisconsin Ave., Milwaukee, WI 53226, USA
[d]Mayo Clinic College of Medicine, Arizona Sports Medicine Center, 5111 N. Scottsdale Road,
Suite 101, Scottsdale, Arizona 85250, USA
[e]Killington Medical Clinic, Vermont Orthopedic Clinic, PO Box 205, Killington, VT, USA

Today's athletes are often unsatisfied with the traditional sports of the past. Even sports that were considered "extreme" in previous generations, such as the marathon, have been made harder by adding length (eg, ultramarathons), by adding events (eg, triathlons), or by placing them in extreme locations (eg, jungles, mountains, or deserts). Other extreme sports are based on activities such as climbing and skateboarding. Physicians taking care of athletes who participate in these sports face a variety of challenges including the exposure of these athletes to unusual infectious diseases [1].

This article discusses infections that may be more likely to occur in the extreme sport athlete, such as selected parasitic infections, marine infections, freshwater-borne diseases, tick-borne disease, and zoonoses. Epidemiology, presentation, treatment, complications, and return-to-sport issues are discussed for each of these diseases.

PARASITES

Parasitic infection can plague athletes traveling to and competing in the developing world. Extreme sport athletes may be at increased risk because they often travel through poorer, rural areas of tropical and subtropical regions to reach their destinations. Risk from a specific parasite depends on the region

*Corresponding author. Department of Orthopaedic Surgery, Medical College of Wisconsin, 9200 W. Wisconsin Ave., Milwaukee, WI 53226. E-mail address: cyoung@mcw.edu (C.C. Young).

0278-5919/07/$ – see front matter
doi:10.1016/j.csm.2007.04.003

of the world traveled, contact with food or water, and whether traveling in rural or urban areas.

Approximately 8% of travelers returning from the developing world require medical treatment during or after travel. Travelers to sub-Saharan Africa, south central Asia, the Caribbean, and Central or South America who have diarrhea are more likely to have a parasitic cause than a bacterial one. Only in Southeast Asia is traveler's diarrhea more likely to be caused be bacteria [2]. Parasitic infection can occur from ingestion of contaminated food and water, from environmental exposure, or from person-to-person or person-to-soil contact. Parasitic illness can be manifest in a variety of ways, depending on the causative organism. A returning traveler who has eosinophilia and fever has a high likelihood of having a parasitic infection. Other common findings include fever, diarrhea, weight loss, neurologic symptoms, dermatologic findings, eosinophilia or other laboratory abnormalities, and ova on stool studies.

Amoebiasis, caused by *Entamoeba histolytica*, is the most common urban gastrointestinal parasite and the second most common parasitic disease worldwide [3]. Up to 90% of people in endemic countries are asymptomatic carriers of amoebiasis. Although typically thought of as a tropical infection, travelers to southern Italy have contracted the illness [4].

Entamoeba histolytica uses proteases to invade intestinal mucosa or to enter the portal circulation, creating hepatic abscess and killing host cells on contact. The diagnosis of amoebiasis is made by finding cysts or trophozoites in stool. Treatment must eliminate the amoebas in tissue and the luminal amoebas to prevent recurrence. Amoebic colitis and liver abscess, if left untreated, can be fatal, and is the second leading cause of death from parasitic infection worldwide [5]. The treatment is with metronidazole or tinidazole followed by iodoquinol or paromomycin [6]. Asymptomatic carriers can be treated with iodoquinol or paromomycin alone.

Fever following travel can indicate malaria infection, the most common cause of undifferentiated fever in travelers to areas endemic for malaria. The *Anopheles* mosquito serves as the vector for malaria transmission, and travelers to endemic areas should use preventive measures such as screens, nets, repellent containing deet (N,N-diethyltoluamide; 30%–35%), and permethrin spray on clothing. Chloroquine, atovaquone proguanil, or mefloquine can be used prophylactically, which decreases the risk of malaria but does not completely preclude infection.

Most patients who have malaria exhibit a regular pattern of fever every 48 to 72 hours. Ninety percent of *Plasmodium falciparum* infections are acquired in sub-Saharan Africa, whereas 70% of *Plasmodium vivax* infections are acquired in Latin America and Asia [7].

When malaria is suspected, blood smears and other appropriate diagnostic laboratory testing should be performed serially as necessary. Those who have severe complications or who have *Plasmodium falciparum* infection often require inpatient treatment for intensive therapy and to address potential anemia, seizure, renal failure, or respiratory distress. Specific treatment depends on the *Plasmodium* species and on antimalarial resistance.

Intestinal nematode, or roundworm, infections such as *Ascaris lumbricoides* (roundworm), *Trichuris trichiura* (whipworm), *Strongyloides stercoralis*, and hookworm can cause serious health problems, most notably malnutrition and diminished capacity for work. Hookworm requires a soil phase as a part of its development, and infection is from soil transmission. The cause of a soil-transmitted helminth disease is variable, with prevalences as high as 69.9% to 100% from a mixture of *Ascaris lumbricoides*, *Trichuris trichiura*, and hookworm in natives of endemic regions [3,8]. Hookworm infection can occur easily, as illustrated by a case when a traveler merely visited a beach in Thailand [9].

Most individuals remain asymptomatic but can exhibit iron deficiency anemia, hypoalbuminemia, and eosinophilia. Delays in appearance of stool ova can make diagnosis of acute hookworm infection difficult, and resistance to empiric treatment with ivermectin can make initial treatment a challenge [10]. Diagnosis is made by detection of eggs or larvae in stool. Treatment is with albendazole or mebendazole.

Strongyloidiasis is caused by the nematode parasite *Strongyloides stercoralis*. Transmission may be from person to person or from contact with soil. Autoinfection can also be a prominent feature of the *Strongyloides* lifecycle [11]. Strongyloidiasis among East African and Cambodian immigrants to Australia is 11% and 42%, respectively [12]. In children living in Papua New Guinea, *Strongyloides* infects 40% in the youngest age group [13].

Infection with *Strongyloides* may be asymptomatic but can progress to disseminated infection or fatal hyperinfection. Symptoms can involve the gastrointestinal system and pulmonary system, or can disseminate to other organ systems. Pulmonary *Strongyloides* infection can lead to a refractory bronchial asthma, cause an acute eosinophilic pneumonia, or can be fulminant and fatal. Arthritis may be associated with *Strongyloides* infection, causing painful, swollen joints. Treatment with nonsteroidal anti-inflammatory drugs can be effective for the symptoms, but corticosteroids can induce a life-threatening *Strongyloides* hyperinfection syndrome, and antihelminth therapy should be given first [14].

Strongyloidiasis can affect athletes traveling to tropical and subtropical regions. Eosinophilia raises suspicion, and diagnosis can be made by detecting eggs or larvae in stool, sputum, pleural fluid, or tissue and confirmed with serologic testing [15]. Even with laboratory testing, diagnosis can be elusive with *Strongyloides*. In a study of people who have microscopically proven *Strongyloides* infection, only 73% of travelers had a positive serology compared with 98% of immigrants from endemic countries. There was no difference with eosinophilia, with 81% in both groups [16]. When established, strongyloidiasis should be treated with ivermectin or albendazole. Local deworming projects in less developed countries have had mixed results, with developing resistance and difficulty with sustainability of the projects making it likely that helminth risk to traveling athletes will remain [17].

Travelers to the tropics can develop cutaneous manifestations that can easily be misdiagnosed. Hookworm can manifest as cutaneous larva migrans (CLM), acquired by skin contact with the soil. Case reports show CLM after a beach vacation to Thailand [18]. Itchy, sleep-disrupting papules typically affect the feet and buttocks and develop into linear or serpiginous red streaks. Larva currens from *Strongyloides stercoralis* can present as an intensely itching wheal in a serpiginous line that progresses 5 to 15 cm/h [18]. Myiasis, whereby larvae invasively feed on living tissue, is traditionally considered a low risk in travelers to tropical areas. Adventure athletes and travelers to the tropics, however, have a higher risk of screwworm infestation [19,20] with increased exposure and the physical duress of competition.

Other parasitic infections to consider in the returning traveling athlete include infections with other protozoa such as *Leishmania*, extraintestinal nematodes such as *Filaria*, cestodes (flat worms), trematodes (flukes) such as *Schistosoma*, and ectoparasites such as lice and scabies. Athletes who travel to tropical and subtropical regions of the world must use preventive measures, and practitioners who care for these athletes at home should be aware of the possibility of parasitic infection and use appropriate diagnostics and treatments.

MARINE INFECTIONS

Although folklore commonly considers seawater an antiseptic, in reality, seawater contains many potential pathogens including *Escherichia coli*, *Pseudomonas aeruginosa*, *Mycobacterium marinum*, *Staphylococcus aureus*, *Streptococcus* species, *Clostridium* species, and *Vibrio* species [21,22]. Thus, even small lacerations and abrasions are at risk for atypical skin infections that have a tendency to be refractory to standard antimicrobial treatment [22].

Marine infections are also common after marine envenomation or fish bites. Many marine fish spines, including those of surgeonfish and stingrays, have spines that break off during the defensive "attack" and result in contamination of the wound with not only a neurotoxic venom but also fragments of the spine, mucus coating, and pieces of the sheath [23]. Coral reef scrapes are also often contaminated with foreign material, various microbes, and toxins from multiple sources [21,24]. These contaminates lead to a high rate of secondary bacterial infection and delayed healing.

All marine-related wounds should be vigorously irrigated and debrided, if necessary. Antibiotics are not usually needed for new and minor wounds unless the victim has an impaired immune system [25]. Because of the relatively high prevalence of atypical pathogens, any significant wound or any nonhealing wound should be cultured before starting antibiotics. In general, ciprofloxacin and trimethoprim-sulfamethoxazole are the best antibiotics for empiric coverage of marine bacteria [25]. Alternative antibiotics include tetracycline and doxycycline. Athletes should be warned about the potential photosensitizing effect of these antibiotics and instructed to take appropriate precautions to limit ultraviolet radiation exposure. Because of the limited access to treatment, athletes participating in multiday adventure races often present for treatment a considerable time after suffering the injury. For these athletes, delayed wound closure should be considered. Although delayed wound closure often leads to a poorer cosmetic result; it is associated with improved wound healing and decreased risk of infection [22]. Another situation in which delayed wound closure should be considered is in the case of a large wound that has been immersed in seawater. In these wounds, early suturing often leads to delayed healing; thus, strong consideration should be given to delayed wound closure unless suturing is needed to protect vital underlying structures [25]. All athletes who have marine wounds need to have an up-to-date tetanus booster because of the high risk of associated *Clostridium* infection.

Many marine wounds (eg, stingray, jellyfish, coral) are accompanied by envenomation. Mild envenomation results predominantly in skin irritation. Severe envenomation may lead to neurologic, respiratory, cardiovascular, musculoskeletal, renal, and gastrointestinal complications or even failure [22–24]. Some of the more severe poisons such as the box-jellyfish and stonefish have commercially available antivenom. In general, avoid using freshwater to rinse off any hydroid (eg, jellyfish) fragments to prevent further nematocyst discharge. Instead, most wilderness medicine authors recommend using a solution composed of 50% acetic acid (5% concentration) and 50% isopropyl alcohol (40%–70% concentration) or seawater [21,24]. Some toxins (eg, stingray) are heat labile, and soaking the wound in nonscalding hot water (up to 45°C/ 113°F) for 30 to 90 minutes may provide some relief. Because systemic symptoms may have a delayed onset of several hours, all athletes who have marine envenomation should be carefully observed for an extended period [24].

FRESHWATER-BORNE DISEASES

Freshwater can also harbor sources of infectious disease for athletes. Athletes often come in contact with water during training and competition, but many do not realize that the development of the host country, the season, and the duration of exposure put them at significant risk for water-borne diseases [2]. Some of the more common water-borne disease threats come from *Giardia, Cryptosporidium,* and *Schistosoma* species.

Giardia lamblia (also known as *Giardia intestinalis* and *Giardia duodenalis*) is a common protozoan parasite that can be found throughout the world [26,27] but has a higher incidence in the summer and autumn and in developing countries located in temperate climates [26–28]. It is one of the most common causes of chronic diarrhea [26,27]. Usually spread by way of the fecal-oral route, the pathogenic mechanism of *Giardia* is believed to be by adherence to the small intestine mucosa through ingestion of cysts in drinking water, food, or recreational surface water or by close person-to-person contact [26–28]. *Giardia* infection can be caused by exposure to as few as 10 to 25 cysts and has an incubation period ranging from 3 to 40 days, with transmission possible for up to 6 months [28]. While 25% to 30% of infected persons are asymptomatic, symptoms commonly include abdominal cramps, foul-smelling and greasy stools, flatulence, bloating, nausea, excessive tiredness, anorexia, and weight loss. Unlike many waterborne diseases, eosinophilia and urticaria are not common findings [27]. Definitive diagnosis is traditionally made by examination of stool for ova and parasite by trichrome iodine staining or by direct immunofluorescence; however, enzyme-linked immunosorbent assay (ELISA) testing is becoming the preferred method [27]. Metronidazole is the treatment of choice, with albendazole as a second line for resistant cases [27]. Symptoms of mild to moderate diarrhea can also be improved with the use of loperamide or bismuth preparations [5]. The cornerstone of prevention, as with any fecal-oral infection, is diligent hand washing and not ingesting anything that has not been fully cooked or peeled.

Cryptosporidium parvum is another protozoan parasite that is a cause of waterborne disease worldwide [27]. Like Giardia, it is more common in developing countries, but because of its resistance to eradication by chlorine and other purification techniques, there continue to be many outbreaks even in industrialized countries [27,29]. Spread by the fecal-oral route, Cryptosporidium infection is often a cause of persistent diarrhea [28]. Although the pathogenic mechanism is unknown, Cryptosporidium is thought to infect the small bowel preferentially [27,28]. There are two genotypes of Cryptosporidium: genotype 1, which causes infection in humans; and genotype 2, which causes infection in animals [27]. Different phenotypes have also recently been demonstrated that affect the severity of symptoms and, therefore, it may take as little as 10 oocysts or as many as 1000 to cause symptomatic disease [27,28]. Infection is through ingestion of cysts in drinking water, food, or recreational surface water or by close person-to-person contact. Symptoms of disease include persistent (>14 days) or chronic (>30 days) watery diarrhea, cramping, abdominal pain, fatigue, nausea, vomiting, occasional low-grade fever, dyspepsia, and asthenia [27,28]. In the past, the diagnosis has been confirmed by acid-fast stain of fecal samples, looking for oocysts or monoclonal-direct immunoassay, but due to the low sensitivity of these traditional techniques, ELISA testing has become the mainstay of laboratory testing [27]. Treatment for Cryptosporidium infection remains symptomatic control with loperamide or bismuth preparations [27,30]. Some studies have shown paromomycin and azithromycin to decrease symptoms and parasitic load, but these medications are not the mainstay of treatment for immunocompetent persons at this time [27].

Schistosomiasis, caused by a helminth parasite, affects more than 200 million people worldwide and is endemic to sub-Saharan Africa, South America, and Southeast Asia [15,31–34]. Three main species cause most of the infections: Schistosoma mansoni and Schistosoma japonicum are responsible for disease affecting the pulmonary system, gastrointestinal tract, or hepatosplenic tract, whereas Schistosoma haematobium usually affects the urinary tract [7,10,12,13]. Humans contract the disease by swimming in freshwater infected with Schistosoma cercaria, which are larvae secreted by the host snail species Biomphalaria glabrata and Biomphalaria straminea [15,31–35]. The infection course follows three stages. Stage 1 consists of an itchy maculopapular rash that is caused by the cercaria penetrating the skin after swimming in infested water and resolves in 48 to

72 hours [7,8,10,12,13]. Stage 2, acute schistosomiasis, occurs 4 to 6 weeks after exposure and is characterized by Katayama fever, a manifestation of the immune-mediated response to the release of the first set of eggs from the mature schistosomes [15,31–34]. Signs and symptoms of Katayama fever are similar to a serum sickness reaction and include fever, malaise, eosinophilia, hepatosplenomegaly, diarrhea, urticaria, edema, cough, wheezing, arthralgias, headache, abdominal pain, lymphadenopathy, and micro- or macrohematuria [15,31–34]. Stage 3, chronic schistosomiasis, results from granulomatous or fibrotic responses (or both) to further egg deposition. Depending on the infecting species and the extent of infection, different manifestations can occur. Chronic infection by *Schistosoma mansoni* and *Schistosoma japonicum* can cause pulmonary fibrosis that can lead to pulmonary hypertension and cor pulmonale, periportal fibrosis, portal hypertension, and portosystemic anastamoses [15,32–34]. In rare cases, central nervous system involvement occurs, with infection of the spinal cord and brain with passage of eggs through the paravertebral venous plexus [31]. Chronic *Schistosoma haematobium* infection can cause urinary granulomas, obstructive uropathy, hydronephrosis, and calcified fibrotic bladder or ureter (or both) [31,36].

Diagnosis of acute schistosomiasis is usually made by correlating the typical signs, symptoms, and exposure history to water in an endemic area and confirmed by eosinophilia and schistosome eggs found in stool or urine [15,31,32]. Diagnosis of chronic schistosomiasis is usually made by antibody detection by ELISA, indirect hemagglutination, and the circuoval precipitin test [31]. Often, exposed travelers will remain asymptomatic, and diagnosis is made years later by CT of the head, chest, or abdomen or by cystoscopy [31,36]. The mainstay of treatment for schistosomiasis is praziquantel [15,31,37]; however, praziquantel is only effective against the adult schistosome. Therefore, repetitive treatment courses may be necessary to prevent reoccurrance [31,37]. Recently, there have been reported cases of resistance to praziquantel. Therefore, close monitoring and documentation of clearance of disease is necessary [36]. Recent research has shown that application of deet before swimming in endemic areas can reduce the risk of contraction of disease [37].

TICK-BORNE DISEASES

Tick-borne diseases potentially pose a threat to athletes who participate in outdoor activities. Ticks can be found throughout the United States, and the diagnosis of tick-borne diseases should be based on the history, clinical presentation, and known epidemiology of the disease. Coinfections are relatively common, with babesiosis occurring in 23% and ehrlichiosis occurring in up to 30% of patients who have Lyme disease [38]. Prophylaxis after a tick bite is generally not recommended, but treatment of suspected disease should not be delayed for laboratory diagnosis in all cases.

Ticks generally require 24 to 48 hours of attachment to transmit disease; they should therefore be removed from the skin as soon as possible. The best way to remove a tick is by grasping the tick as close to the skin as possible with tweezers or a hand and gently pulling with straight traction. Avoid squeezing the body during tick removal because this theoretically may cause the tick to regurgitate its stomach contents, thereby increasing the risk of disease. Avoid twisting the tick because this may result in the breaking off of mouthparts. Do not apply anything such as petroleum jelly, gasoline, or heat to the tick because none of these methods have proved effective in detaching the tick and may increase the risk of disease transmission. After tick removal, monitor the attachment sites for any signs of infection [39].

Prevention is best accomplished by applying a deet-containing repellent before outdoor activities. Other helpful measures include wearing long-sleeved and long-legged clothing and body examination after being in the outdoors [40].

Although there have been no specific reports of outbreaks of tick-borne disease during athletic events, athletes have similar risks to others participating in outdoor activities in endemic areas. Return-to-play decisions should be based on the same factors one would use for other illnesses. Because many tick-borne diseases present with an influenza-like syndrome, absence of fever and resolution of malaise and fatigue are the main criteria for return to activity.

Lyme disease is the most common vector-borne infectious disease in the United States [38,41]. It can be found throughout the United States, but is most commonly reported in endemic areas: the coastal Northeast and parts of the upper Midwest. *Borrelia burgdorferi* is the spirochete that causes the infection. There are typically three stages of Lyme disease. Stage 1, early localized, occurs 7 to 10 days after a tick bite. Three fourths of patients develop the characteristic rash, erythema migrans, at the site of the tick bite. The rash is an annular macule or papule with central clearing. Infected persons commonly experience influenza-like symptoms with low-grade fevers, fatigue, arthralgias, headaches, cough, and lymphadenopathy. Symptoms of stage 2, early disseminated, include secondary skin lesions, adenopathy, and central nervous system symptoms. These symptoms typically occur within a few weeks of the initial infection. Stage 3, late chronic disease, may present with arthritis, dermatitis, keratitis, Bell's palsy, meningoencephalitis, and myocardial abnormalities [38,41].

It is important to recognize endemic versus nonendemic areas when diagnosing Lyme disease. Patients from endemic areas who present with erythema migrans should be treated, and no laboratory testing is required. For patients in nonendemic areas who have unclear symptoms, ELISA testing can be used with reasonable sensitivity (89%) but relatively poor specificity (72%). Positive ELISA test should be confirmed with Western blot testing. Routine testing is not recommended after a tick bite [42].

The overall risk of infection after a tick bite is very low and almost never occurs unless the tick has been attached at least 36 hours. This is true even for endemic areas. Prophylaxis with one 200-mg dose of doxycycline is effective but not routinely recommended. Patients who sustain a tick bite should be monitored for up to 30 days post bite [41,42]. For those who develop symptoms, antibiotic treatment is curative in most cases. Two to 3 weeks of treatment with doxycycline (100 mg twice per day) or amoxicillin (500 mg three times per day) is generally effective for adults. Patients who have severe or late disease may require hospitalization and intravenous antibiotics [41–43].

Return to play for uncomplicated Lyme disease should be based on resolution of clinical symptoms. Late disease, especially with cardiac complications or arthritis, should be guided by consultation with a specialist and may require several months out of competition.

Rocky Mountain spotted fever (RMSF) is caused by *Rickettsia rickettsii* and is the most common rickettsial disease in the United States [43]. RMSF is a misnomer because this disease is found most commonly in the Atlantic eastern states. RMSF has been reported in all states except Maine, Alaska, and Hawaii. The highest infection rates are in young children. Most people infected remember having a tick bite, and symptoms generally start 5 to 7 days after inoculation. Classic presentation includes an acute onset of fever, chills, and headache, with the onset of a rash in the first few days. Lesions first appear on the palms, soles, wrists, ankles, and forearms and then extend over the trunk, buttock, and face. The rash is initially maculopapular but becomes more petechial as the disease progresses [38,43].

Diagnosis is based primarily on clinical signs and symptoms. Laboratory testing has limited use. Skin biopsy of the rash using immunofluorescent staining is relatively specific but has low sensitivity. Complete blood count is generally normal. Mild elevations in liver enzyme levels and thrombocytopenia are sometimes found [38].

Human monocytic ehrlichiosis (HME), caused by *Ehrlichia chaffeensis,* and human granulocytotropic anaplasmosis (HGA), formerly human granulocytic ehrlichiosis, caused by *Anaplasma phagocytophilum*, are epidemiologically separate but clinically indistinguishable [38,43]. HME is generally found in the south-central and southeastern United States, whereas HGA occurs in the upper Midwest and northeastern United States.

It can be difficult to distinguish between the clinical presentation of ehrlichiosis and RMSF [38,43]. Signs and symptoms of *Ehrlichia* infection include an influenza-like syndrome and generally begin 7 days after the tick bite. In addition to fever, chills, malaise, cough, headache, and myalgias, an infected person may develop a maculopapular, macular, or petechial rash. This rash differs from the rash of RMSF because it rarely (<5%) affects the palms and soles. Laboratory findings may include leukopenia, thrombocytopenia, and elevated liver enzymes. Confirmation of the diagnosis of ehrlichiosis may be detected by seroconversion [38,43].

Treatment and return to activity after infection with *Rickettsia, Ehrlichia,* or *Anaplasma* are similar. Antibiotics should be started as soon as a clinical suspicion is raised and should not be delayed for laboratory testing. Doxycycline, 100 mg twice a day for adults or 2.2 mg/kg for children, is the first-line drug. No clear guidelines exist for duration of treatment, but antibiotics should be continue for at least 3 days after fever resolves, usually 5 to 7 days minimum [38]. Chloramphenicol is an alternative treatment, but its use is limited by potential toxicity. Return to play after treatment should not be considered until clinical symptoms resolve.

Babesiosis most often occurs in the northeastern United States and is the only tick-borne disease caused by a protozoan in this country [43]. Symptoms include fever, sweating, myalgias, and headache. Laboratory findings include hemolytic anemia, hemoglobinuria, and in severe cases, jaundice and renal failure. Peripheral smear will sometimes demonstrate organisms within erythrocytes. The diagnosis is generally made by blood smears, although serologic and polymerase chain reaction testing is available [44].

Symptomatic treatment is recommended for mild disease. For patients who have severe symptoms such as persistent high fever and progressive anemia, quinine (650 mg) and clindamycin (600 mg) three times a day for 7 days is recommended. Alternative treatments include atovaquone and azythromycin [44]. For mild disease, return to activity may start as symptoms and anemia improve. Athletes who have severe cases should be monitored closely and not start activity until anemia, fevers, and any renal complications have resolved.

ZOONOSES

Zoonoses are animal diseases that are transmissible to humans. Humans generally acquire the disease through close contact with an infected animal. Routes of transmission include infectious saliva from bite wounds; aerosol from body fluids (especially respiratory); scratches; hand-to-mouth transmission of microorganisms, cysts, or oocysts from infected animal feces; insect bites when the insect is acting as a reservoir between the animal and humans; and contamination of water or the environment with disease-containing animal urine.

Leptospirosis is a zoonosis with protean manifestations caused by the spirochete *Leptospira interrogans*. Synonyms for the disease include Weil's disease, swineherd's disease, rice-field fever, cane-cutter fever, swamp fever, mud fever, hemorrhagic jaundice, Stuttgart disease, and canicola fever. The organism infects a variety of mammals, especially rodents, cattle, swine, dogs, horses, sheep, and goats. When infected, animals may shed the organism in their urine intermittently or continuously throughout life [45]. Organisms may remain viable for days to months in soil and water, and humans most often become infected after exposure to freshwater contaminated by rodent urine [46]. Portals of entry include cuts or abraded skin, mucous membranes, or conjunctiva. In the United States, most cases are reported from the southern and Pacific coastal states, with Hawaii consistently reporting the most cases. Most clinical cases occur in the tropics [47,48], and the incidence of leptospirosis in some endemic countries appears to be increasing, with Thailand reporting a 30-fold increase between 1995 and 2000, possibly due to an increase in the rat population [49].

Outbreaks may occur from common-source exposures. Participation in a triathlon where the swimming portion was in contaminated freshwater has been found to be responsible for outbreaks of leptospirosis. An outbreak occurred in

98 of 834 athletes (12%) participating in an Illinois triathlon [50]. Another recent outbreak among athletes participating in the "Eco-Challenge Sabah 2000" competition occurred in Borneo, Malaysia. The athletes presented with fever, jaundice, headache, and myalgias after returning home, and 44% of 158 athletes contacted met the case definition [51].

Leptospirosis is associated with a variable clinical course. The disease may manifest as a subclinical illness followed by seroconversion, a self-limited systemic infection, or a severe, potentially fatal illness accompanied by multiorgan failure. Leptospirosis presents with the abrupt onset of fever, rigors, myalgias, and headache in 75% to 100% of patients. Although leptospirosis has often been described as a biphasic illness, less than 50% of cases exhibit a biphasic course [47]. Most cases of leptospirosis are mild to moderate; however, the course may be complicated by renal failure, uveitis, hemorrhage, acute respiratory distress syndrome, myocarditis, and rhabdomyolysis [52]. The clinical features and routine laboratory findings of leptospirosis are not specific. The organism can be cultured, but the diagnosis is more frequently made by serologic testing [53].

Although most *Leptospira* infections are self-limiting, antimicrobial treatment results in a shorter duration of illness. Doxycycline and penicillin have been shown to be effective in placebo-controlled trials [54]. Parenteral penicillin, doxycycline, and third-generation cephalosporins are acceptable options in hospitalized patients, although in areas endemic for leptospirosis and rickettsial infection, a regimen other than penicillin should be considered [55]. Mortality rates in hospitalized patients who have leptospirosis have ranged from 4% to 52%, with higher mortality rates occurring in patients requiring ICU admission on presentation [56]. No vaccine is available in the United States for human immunization. The major preventive measure is to avoid potential sources of infection. Consider prophylaxis with doxycycline (200 mg/wk) for individuals such as river rafters and swimmers who will be exposed to leptospires in highly endemic environments [57].

Hantaviruses compose a genus of enveloped viruses within the family Bunyaviridae. These pathogens are associated with two severe, acute febrile illnesses: hemorrhagic fever with renal syndrome (HFRS) in Europe and Asia and hantavirus cardiopulmonary syndrome, also known as hantavirus pulmonary syndrome (HPS), in the Americas.

Each hantavirus is specifically associated with a single species of wild rodent, which serves as its primary natural reservoir. The deer mouse is the primary vector in the United States [58]. The incidence of hantavirus infections in humans fluctuates with rodent densities [59]. Hantaviruses are shed in the urine, feces, or saliva of acutely infected reservoir rodents, and transmission to humans generally occurs by way of the aerosol route [60]. Athletes who compete in outdoor activities in wilderness areas or who camp are at higher risk of exposure.

HFRS first came to the attention of Western medicine during the Korean War, when febrile illness accompanied by hemorrhage and renal failure developed in 3000 United Nations soldiers [61]. HFRS has a variable incubation period and is characterized by five phases. The initial febrile phase lasts 3 to 7 days and is characterized by fever, malaise, headache, abdominal pain, nausea, vomiting, facial flushing, petechiae, and conjunctival hemorrhage. A hypotensive phase follows, which can lead to shock, blurred vision, and hemorrhagic signs. An oliguric phase lasting 3 to 7 days is followed by a diuretic phase lasting days to weeks. The complete convalescence may take weeks to months. Mortality resulting from shock, uremia, or multiorgan hypoperfusion occurs in 1% to 10% [58]. Early treatment with ribavirin may reduce hemorrhage, renal failure, and mortality in HFRS [62].

HPS was discovered in 1993, when a series of cases of unexplained fever and acute respiratory distress syndrome was recognized among members of the Navajo tribe at the northern border between New Mexico and Arizona [63]. The mortality rate was approximately 80% in the initial patients.

The clinical progression of HPS advances through four sequential stages. Typically, a period of 3 weeks elapses between exposure to a hantavirus and the first symptoms [64,65]. The febrile stage typically lasts 3 to 5 days and is characterized by fever, myalgias, and malaise. This stage is difficult to distinguish from a number of nonspecific viral syndromes. The disease rapidly increases in severity, often leading to nausea, vomiting, abdominal pain, weakness, and sometimes diarrhea and headache. Classic features of upper respiratory tract infection such as rhinorrhea, pharyngitis, coryza, and ear pain are absent in most patients who have hantavirus diseases. The simultaneous appearance of thrombocytopenia, a left-shifted granulocytic series, and an immunoblast count that exceeds 10% of the total lymphoid series is referred to as the diagnostic triad [60]. A dry cough often heralds the sudden transition to the cardiopulmonary phase [63], which is characterized by shock and pulmonary edema [66,67]. Hypoxia and circulatory compromise often lead to death. The pulmonary edema clears during the diuretic phase, and fever resolves [60]. Complete recovery generally occurs but can take months [68]. Serologic tests are the main method for diagnosis of acute or remote infection by hantaviruses.

Treatment of HPS is supportive. Early recognition, hospitalization, and adequate pulmonary and hemodynamic support in an intensive care setting are important. No specific antiviral therapy for HPS is available [62]. Given the limited treatment options and high mortality rates, emphasis needs to be on avoidance of exposure to potentially infectious rodents, particularly in indoor spaces.

PREVENTION AND MEDICAL EVENT COVERAGE

Because of the nature of their sports, the use of protective clothing and sleeping areas by extreme athletes is usually limited. Thus, the use of insect repellent is particularly important. Athletes should be encouraged to avoid untreated water for hydration and told to carry water purification tablets in their required first aid supplies. Because many of the extreme sport events take place in relatively isolated locations, it is essential that medical coverage planning include transportation and evacuation routes. For events in overseas locations, it is recommended that all competitors have insurance that covers evacuation by helicopter or fixed-wing aircraft because often, operators of medical evacuation services will refuse to fly until they have proof of payment [69].

SUMMARY

Extreme sport competition often takes place in locations that may harbor atypical diseases. The lack of immediate medical care can complicate and worsen the severity of these diseases. Physicians caring for extreme sport competitors must take a careful travel and exposure history and have a high index of suspicion for unusual diseases.

References

[1] Young C. Extreme sports: injuries and medical coverage. Curr Sports Med Rep 2002;1(5): 306–11.

[2] Freedman D, Weld L, Kozarsky P. Spectrum of disease and relation to place of exposure among ill returned travelers. N Engl J Med 2006;354(2):119–30.

[3] Abd El Bagi M, Sammak B, Mohamed A, et al. Gastrointestinal parasite infestation. Eur Radiol 2004;14(Suppl 3):E116–31.

[4] Edeling W, Verweij J, Ponsioen C, et al. Outbreak of amoebiasis in a Dutch family; tropics unexpectedly nearby. Ned Tijdschr Geneeskd 2004;148(37):1830–4.

[5] Stanley SJ. Amoebiasis. Lancet 2003;361(9362):1025–34.

[6] Kitchen L. Case studies in international travelers. Am Fam Physician 1999;60(2):471–4.

[7] Ryan E, Wilson M, Kain K. Illness after international travel. N Engl J Med 2002;347: 505–16.

[8] Al-Mekhlafi M, Azlin M, Nor Aini U, et al. Prevalence and distribution of soil-transmitted helminthiases among Orang Asli children living in peripheral Selangor, Malaysia, Southeast Asia. J Trop Med Public Health 2006;37(1):40–7.

[9] Malvy D, Ezzedine K, Pistone T, et al. Extensive cutaneous larva migrans with folliculitis mimicking multimetameric Herpes Zoster presentation in an adult traveler returning from Thailand. J Travel Med 2006;13(4):244–7.

[10] Lawn S, Grant A, Wright S. Case reports: acute hookworm infection: an unusual cause of profuse watery diarrhoea in returned travelers. Trans R Soc Trop Med Hyg 2003;97(4): 414–5.

[11] Vadlamudi R, Chi D, Krishnaswamy G. Intestinal strongyloidiasis and hyperinfection syndrome. Clin Mol Allergy 2006;4:8.

[12] Caruana S, Kelly H, Ngeow J, et al. Undiagnosed and potentially lethal parasite infections among immigrants and refugees in Australia. J Travel Med 2006;13(4):233–4.

[13] Barnish G, Ashford R. *Strongyloides cf. Fuelleborni* and hookworm in Papua New Guinea: patterns of infection within the community. Trans R Soc Trop Med Hyg 1989;83(5):684–8.

[14] Richter J, Muller-Stover I, Strothmeyer H, et al. Arthritis associated with *Strongyloides stercoralis* infection in a HLA B-27-positive African. Parasitol Res 2006;99(6):706–7.

[15] Kuzucu A. Parasitic diseases of the respiratory tract. Curr Opin Pulm Med 2006;12(3): 212–21.

[16] Sudarshi S, Stumpfle R, Armstrong M, et al. Clinical presentation and diagnostic sensitivity of laboratory tests for *Strongyloides stercoralis* in travelers compared with immigrants in a non-endemic country. Trop Med Int Health 2003;8(8):728–32.

[17] Bethony J, Brooker S, Albonico M. Soil-transmitted helminth infections: ascariasis, trichuriasis, and hookworm. Lancet 2006;367(9521):1521–32.

[18] Wolf R, Marcos B, Orion E, et al. Widespread pruritic papulopustules after returning from Thailand. Am Fam Physician 2005;72(11):2313–4.

[19] Seppanen M, Virolainen-Julkunen A, Kakko I, et al. Myiasis during adventure sports race. Emerg Infect Dis 2004;10(1):137–9.

[20] Siraj D, Luczkovich J. Nodular skin lesion in a returning traveler. J Travel Med 2005;12(4): 229–31.

[21] Zoltan T, Taylor K. Health issues for surfers. Am Fam Physician 2005;71(12):2313–7.

[22] Auerbach P, Halstead B. Injuries from nonvenomous aquatic animals. In: Auerbach P, editor. Wilderness medicine. 4th edition. St. Louis (MO): Mosby; 2001. p. 1418–49.

[23] Auerbach P. Envenomation by aquatic vertebrates. In: Auerbach P, editor. Wilderness medicine. 4th edition. St. Louis (MO): Mosby; 2001. p. 1488–506.

[24] Auerbach P. Envenomation by aquatic invertebrates. In: Auerbach P, editor. Wilderness medicine. 4th edition. St. Louis (MO): Mosby; 2001. p. 1450–87.

[25] Auerbach P. A medical guide to hazardous marine life. 3rd edition. Flagstaff (AZ): Dive Alert Network; 1997.

[26] Ekdahl K, Anderson Y. Imported giardiasis: impact of international travel, immigration, and adoption. Am J Tropical Med 2005;72(6):825–30.

[27] Okhuysen P. Traveler's diarrhea due to intestinal protoza. Clin Infect Dis 2001;33:110–4.

[28] Gascon J. Epidemiology, etiology and pathophysiology of traveler's diarrhea. Digestion 2006;73:102–8.

[29] Mathieu E, Levy D, Veverka F, et al. Epidemiologic and environmental investigation of a recreational water outbreak caused by two genotypes of Cryptosporidium parvum in Ohio in 2000. Am J Tropical Med 2004;71(5):582–9.

[30] Aldo A. Tropical diarrhoea: new developments in traveller's diarrhoea. Curr Opin Infect Dis 2001;14:547–52.

[31] Corachan M. Schistosomiasis and international travel. Clin Infect Dis 2001;35:446–50.

[32] Moore E, Doherty J. Schistosomiasis among travellers returning from Malawi: a common occurrence. QJM 2005;98:69–71.

[33] Nguyen L, Estrella J, Jett E, et al. Acute schistosomiasis in nonimmune travelers: chest CT findings in 10 patients. AJR Am J Roentgenol 2006;186:1300–3.

[34] Salanitri J, Stanley P, Hennessy O. Acute pulmonary schistosomiasis. Australas Radiol 2002;46:435–7.

[35] Enk M, Caldeira R, Carvalho O, et al. Rural tourism as risk factors for the transmission of schistosomiasis in Minas Gerais, Brazil. Scielo Brazil 2004;99(1):105–8.

[36] Silva IM, Thiengo R, Conceicao MJ, et al. Cystoscopy in the diagnosis and follow-up of urinary schistosomiasis in Brazilian soldiers returning from Mozambique. Africa Rev Inst Med Trop S Paulo 2006;48(1):39–42.

[37] Jackson F, Doherty J, Beherns R. Schistosomiasis prophylaxis in vivo using N,N-diethyl-m-toluamide (DEET). Trans R Soc Trop Med 2003;97(4):449–50.

[38] Chapman A, Bakken J, Folk S, et al. Diagnosis and management of tick-borne rickettsial diseases: Rocky Mountain spotted fever, ehrlichiosis, and anaplasmosis—United States: a practical guide for physicians and other health-care and public health professionals. MMWR Recomm Rep 2006;55(RR-4):1–27.

[39] Gammons M, Salam G. Tick removal. Am Fam Physician 2002;66:643–5.

[40] Wilson M. Prevention of tick-borne diseases. Med Clin North Am 2002;86:219–38.

[41] Wormser G. Early Lyme disease. N Engl J Med 2006;354:2794–801.

[42] Wormser G, Nadelman R, Dattwyler R, et al. Practice guidelines for the treatment of Lyme disease. Clin Infect Dis 2000;31(Suppl 1):S1–14.

[43] Bratton R, Corey G. Tick-borne disease. Am Fam Physician 2005;71:2323–30.

[44] Homer M, Aguilar-Delfin I, Telford S, et al. Babesiosis. Clin Microbial Rev 2000;13: 451–69.

[45] Acha P, Szyfres B. Leptospirosis. Zoonoses and communicable disease common to man and animals. Washington, DC: 3rd Pan American Health Organization; 2001. p. 157.

[46] Kaufmann A, Weyant R. Leptospiraceae. Manual of clinical microbiology. 6th edition. Washington, DC: ASM Press; 1995. p. 621.

[47] Bertherat E, Renaut A, Nabias R, et al. Leptospirosis and Ebola virus infection in five gold-panning villages in northeastern Gabon. Am J Trop Med Hyg 1999;60:610–5.

[48] Bovet P, Yersin C, Merien F, et al. Factors associated with clinical leptospirosis: a population-based case-control study in the Seychelles (Indian Ocean). Int J Epidemiol 1999;28: 583–90.

[49] Sejvar J, Tangkanakul W, Ratanasang P, et al. An outbreak of leptospirosis, Thailand—the importance of the laboratory. Southeast Asian J Trop Med Public Health 2005;36:289–95.

[50] Morgan J, Bornstein S, Karpati A, et al. Outbreak of leptospirosis among triathlon partici-pants and community residents in Springfield, Illinois, 1998. Clin Infect Dis 2002; 34(12):1593–9.

[51] Centers for Disease Control and Prevention. Update: outbreak of acute febrile illness among athletes participating in Eco-Challenge-Sabah 2000—Borneo, Malaysia, 2000. MMWR 2000;49(36):816–7.

[52] Katz A, Ansdell V, Effler P, et al. Assessment of the clinical presentation and treatment of 353 cases of laboratory-confirmed leptospirosis in Hawaii, 1974–1998. Clin Infect Dis 2001;33(11):1834–41.

[53] Levett P. Usefulness of serologic analysis as a predictor of the infecting serovar in patients with severe leptospirosis. Clin Infect Dis 2003;35(4):447–52.

[54] McClain J, Ballou W, Harrison S, et al. Doxycycline therapy for leptospirosis. Ann Intern Med 1984;100(5):696–8.

[55] Suputtamongkol Y, Niwattayakul K, Suttinont C, et al. An open, randomized, controlled trial of penicillin, doxycycline, and cefotaxime for patients with severe leptospirosis. Clin Infect Dis 2004;39(10):1417–24.

[56] Stefos A, Georgiadou S, Gioti C, et al. Leptospirosis and pancytopenia: two case reports and review of the literature. J Infect 2005;51(5):e277–80.

[57] Takafuji E, Kirkpatrick J, Miller R, et al. An efficacy trial of doxycycline chemoprophylaxis against leptospirosis. N Engl J Med 1984;310(8):497–500.

[58] Glass G. Hantaviruses. Curr Opin Infect Dis 1997;10:362.

[59] Hjelle B, Glass G. Outbreak of hantavirus infection in the Four Corners region of the United States in the wake of the 1997-1998 El Nino-southern oscillation. J Infect Dis 2000;181(5): 1569–73.

[60] Schmaljohn C, Hjelle B. Hantaviruses: a global disease problem. Emerg Infect Dis 1997;3(2):95–104.

[61] Sheedy J, Froeb H, Batson H, et al. The clinical course of epidemic hemorrhagic fever. Am J Med 1954;16(5):619–28.

[62] Peters C, Khan A. Hantavirus pulmonary syndrome: the new American hemorrhagic fever. Clin Infect Dis 2002;34(9):1224–31.

[63] Centers for Disease Control and Prevention. Infectious diseases update: outbreak, hantavi-rus infection—southwestern United States, 1993. JAMA 1993;270(3):306.

[64] Leduc J, Smith G, Johnson K. Hantaan-like viruses from domestic rats captured in the United States. Am J Trop Med Hyg 1984;33(5):992–8.

[65] Lee P, Goldgaber D, Gibbs CJ, et al. Other serotypes of hemorrhagic fever with renal syndrome viruses in Europe. Lancet 1982;2(8312):1405–6.

[66] Jenison S, Hjelle B, Simpson S, et al. Hantavirus pulmonary syndrome: clinical, diagnostic and virologic aspects. Semin Respir Infect 1995;10(4):259–69.

[67] Nichol S, Spirpoulou C, Morzunov S, et al. Genetic identification of a hantavirus associated with an outbreak of acute respiratory illness. Science 1993;262(5135):914–7.

[68] Duchin J, Koster F, Peters C, et al. Hantavirus pulmonary syndrome: a clinical description of 17 patients with a newly recognized disease. The Hantavirus Study Group. N Engl J Med 1994;330(14):949–55.

[69] Mark B. Off the beaten path: rollover in the Namib desert. J Wilderness Med 2006;23(3): 4–8.

ELSEVIER
SAUNDERS

Clin Sports Med 26 (2007) 489–503

CLINICS IN SPORTS MEDICINE

Travel Medicine and the International Athlete

Joel M. Kary, MD[a],*, Mark Lavallee, MD, CSCS, FACSM[a,b,c]

[a]South Bend Sports Medicine Fellowship, Memorial Sports Medicine Institute,
111 West Jefferson Blvd., Suite 100, South Bend, IN 46601, USA
[b]Sports Medicine Committee, USA Weightlifting, US Olympic Training Center,
1 Olympic Plaza, Colorado Springs, CO, USA
[c]International Weightlifting Federation–Masters Program, Budapest, Hungary

M odern sports—professional and amateur—require frequent travel for competition and training. Sports such as American football, baseball, and basketball consist of numerous intracontinental trips, with large contingents of support staff and fans. International travel is common among golfers, track and field athletes, tennis players, and racecar drivers. The summer and winter Olympic Games, Paralympic Games, Commonwealth Games, Pan-Am Games, and World Masters Games, which occur every four years, necessitate international trips. In addition, as recreational sports have increased in popularity, many people are traveling abroad for marathons, triathlons, golf, water sports, and downhill skiing.

Regardless of level of competition (recreational, amateur, or professional), these athletes are confronted with obstacles to optimal performance by the nature of international travel. Furthermore, the coaches, medical team, and staff face challenges of their own in providing support while traveling and working in unfamiliar places. A thoughtful, well-designed plan that addresses issues relating to travel preparation, travel, competition, and post competition allows for an enjoyable and successful experience for the athlete and medical team.

TRAVEL PREPARATION

Before international travel, it is crucial to be well prepared so as to lessen the physical and psychologic stresses that may occur during travel. Preparation for the medical team should begin early, with appropriate selection of team members. The head physician should be experienced at providing medical care during international competitions, well trained in sports medicine, and adept at managing a team of medical caregivers. Selection of the medical team should be guided by the head physician and may vary depending on the type of competition, location, number of athletes, and level of medical care provided at the

*Corresponding author. E-mail address: jmkary1@yahoo.com (J.M. Kary).

0278-5919/07/$ – see front matter
doi:10.1016/j.csm.2007.04.009

competition site. Travel to a developed country with established medical care at smaller competitions may decrease the need for multiple physicians, whereas travel to less developed countries for an event with a large number of athletes may require a larger medical team consisting of multiple physicians and medical volunteers. These medical volunteers may include certified athletic trainers (ATCs), paramedics, Red Cross volunteers, nurses, massage therapists, and chiropractors. The duties and expectations for each member should be clearly delineated and discussed before travel. Team members who are infinitely flexible and willing to help in any capacity, within reason and level of training, can be invaluable to making the experience more enjoyable. A medical team handbook that reviews pertinent issues should be provided. It is very important to be sure that proper licensure and malfeasance insurance is in place for all specialists and that documentation of this is included with travel documents. When care of athletes from other countries is part of the responsibility of the medical team covering the competition while abroad, it is a good idea to obtain guest or temporary medical licensure with the host country. Passports and visas should be obtained well ahead of travel dates and kept current.

Screening physical examinations should be performed for athletes, medical staff, coaches, and support staff before travel. Pertinent past medical history and immunizations should be reviewed in addition to a physical and dental examination, which helps to establish the team member's fitness for duty and ability to comply with the demands of international travel. This review can help identify medical problems that may be problematic during travel and competition, including travel anxiety, asthma, dental caries, gastrointestinal issues, environmental allergies, diabetes, and coronary artery disease. All medical information for traveling team members should be kept secure yet accessible during travel, which can be done by having the head physician carry copies of all medical information in secure carry-on luggage, not in checked luggage.

Mass gatherings such as large sporting events have been associated with outbreaks of infectious disease [1–4]. All athletes and team members should have up-to-date vaccination for tetanus, diphtheria, pertussis, measles, mumps, rubella, and polio [5]. Medical team members and close-contact sports athletes such as boxers, martial artists, and wrestlers should be vaccinated for hepatitis B in a three-dose series [1,6]. Hepatitis A vaccination is usually recommended for all international travelers, especially to developing countries [5]. Athletes who have never had chickenpox or have never been given varicella vaccine should be vaccinated for varicella with two doses 4 to 8 weeks apart [5]. In addition, it may be wise to vaccinate for meningococcal disease and influenza because of cramped living conditions, air travel, and high training loads experienced by athletes. Any further vaccinations such as rabies, typhoid, yellow fever, malaria, cholera, and Japanese encephalitis are recommended depending on the geographic region being visited and the time of year. Comprehensive recommendations for vaccination can be found on the Internet at the Centers for Disease Control and Prevention (www.cdc.gov) and World Health Organization (www.who.int) sites. Education should also be provided to athletes, coaches, and staff on ways to prevent infectious disease while traveling. Prevention methods include washing hands with soap and water or using alcohol-based hand gel, drinking bottled or purified water, eating fully cooked foods, washing or peeling fruits and vegetables before eating, and using abstinence or condoms to avoid sexually transmitted infections [1,5].

Determining the necessary supplies and equipment to bring for international competitions can be challenging, but the following recommendations can help to clarify what is needed. First, no matter what previous arrangements have been made, it may be best to assume that nothing will be provided. Second, the teams should try to be self-sufficient [7]. Third, every effort should be made to communicate ahead of time with the host venue or medical staff. For example, it is important to know whether electricity, water, telephones, the Internet, ice, examination tables, or towels will be provided. Knowing what will be provided in addition to the size, location, and type of competition will help determine what the medical kit should contain. Fig. 1 details the contents of an example medical kit that could be modified for a variety of competitions [8]. A hard-sided medical kit (Fig. 2) withstands the rigors of international travel, transports easily through airports, and allows for convenient organization of medical supplies. A list of all contents in the medical kit should be included with the kit. It would also be appropriate for the head physician to carry a copy of this list to ease transportation of the kit through customs and airports. Medications should be labeled and in appropriate containers. Fig. 3 is a list of suggested medications. For athletes traveling without medical support, a travel health kit is advisable; one is outlined on the Centers for Disease Control and Prevention Web site (www.cdc.gov/travel) (Fig. 4). A travel health kit includes items such as antidiarrheal medication, antiseptic hand gel, a thermometer, and other first aid items [5]. All prescribed medications should be accompanied by a doctor's letter or a copy of the original prescription, along with being contained in original containers [6].

Medical records are important for documentation and medicolegal purposes. If possible, all athletes under medical care should have a health history completed to aid in appropriate diagnosis and treatment of injuries or medical complaints. A medical health history can be difficult to obtain when providing medical coverage for an international event in which the athletes under medical care are from various countries. The authors have created and used an emergency medical form for international weightlifting events that is distributed to all athletes by way of the competition's organizing committee in the athlete's registration packet before the event (Fig. 5). Athletes are instructed to complete and return these forms with their registration by mail or to deliver them at check-in at the event venue. Instructions accompanying the forms request that they be completed in the native language of the medical team to facilitate optimal medical care. An injury report form (Fig. 6) is also used during competition to record all medical encounters, and copies are included with the medical kit or medical team handbook.

Adequate preparation of athletes, coaches, medical team members, and staff includes investigating the political situation of the country being visited for the

Top Tray
Gloves
Screwdriver
Bandage Scissors
Thermometer (Covers)
Tape Measure
Nail Clippers
Safety Pins
Rubber Bands
Batteries
Ammonia Inhalants
Med Dispensing Envelopes
Business Cards
Alcohol preps
Bandages
Antibiotic ointment
Povidone-iodine
Mouthpiece
Assorted athletic tape
Eye Wash
Contact Cleaning Solution
Contact Case
Pen Light
Pocket Mirror
Eye Drops- Isopto Homatropine
Eye Drops- Tetracaine Hydrochloride
Fluoroscein Strips
Albuterol Inhaler
Meds - Naproxen 500 mg
           Ibuprofen 600 mg
           Acetominophen 500 mg
           Chewable Aspirin 81 mg

Middle Tray
Creams-Bactroban Ointment
           Clotrimazole Cream
           Glycerin Lotion
           Muscle Rub
           Triamcinole
           Xylocaine Jelly
           KY Jelly
Swab/Sticks- Benzoin Tincture
           Cotton Tip Applicators
           Ear Curette
           Silver Nitrate Sticks
           Tongue Depressors
Bandage/Wrap- Ace Wraps
           3" Conforming
Laceration Kit -4-0 Ethilon
           4-0 Chromic Gut
           5-0 Ethilon
           Steri Strips ¼ X3
           Steri Strips ½ X4
           Skin Stapler
           Dermabond
           Benzoin Tincture
           Butterfly Bandages
Dressing-   Transparent Adhesive
           Non-Transparent Adhesive
           Non-Adherent Dressing
           Blister Pads
           Gauze Pads
           Moleskin
Bandage- Bandaids
           Finger Bandages
           Nasal Packing
Excision- Scalpel #11, #15
           Surgical Blades
           #10,#11,#15
           Alcohol Preps
           Benzoin Tincture
Instruments- Forceps X 2
           Hemostats – curved
           Hemostats – noncurved
           Scissors
Misc.-   Stethoscope
           BP Cuff
           Sterile Gloves
           Fluro-Meth
           Peroxide
           Pepto Bismol
           Optho/Otoscope
           Slings

Needle/Syringe- 18G,23G, 25G
           3cc, 5cc, 10cc

Lower Tray
Automatic External Defibrillator
CPR Bag/Mask
Pocket Mask
Laryngoscope
Endo Tracheal Tube
Oral Airways
Peak Flow w/ Mouthpieces
Suction device
Sterile Gloves
Sterile Drape
Fiberglass Splints
Sam Splint
Elastic Wraps
Sharps Container
Rescue Blanket
IV Tubing/IV Caths (20G & 22G)
IV Bags – Sodium Chloride 500mL
Bottles- Sodium Chloride
           Sterile Water
Dextrose
Aluminum Finger Splints
DEA/License Papers

Fig. 1. Medical kit contents.

competition. If traveling from the United States, the US Department of State Web site (http://travel.state.gov/) can provide information about conditions abroad that may affect travel safety and security [5]. Other countries may provide the same information by way of their respective government Web sites. Weather forecasts should be reviewed before departure. Acclimatization may be necessary for athletes traveling to high altitudes; hot, humid areas; or cold regions [7,9]. Appropriate apparel should be chosen to allow for comfortable and successful competition.

TRAVEL

Long-distance air travel can cause significant physical and psychologic stress [7,9–16]. Stressors can be related to difficult flight schedules, precompetition

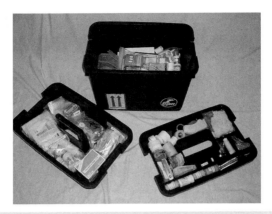

Fig. 2. Medical kit.

anxiety, jet lag, poor sleep, hydration and food concerns, and culture shock on arrival. Strategies to ameliorate these concerns should be discussed and planned before travel.

Athletes and the medical team should arrive early to the airport to allow plenty of time for check in and any extra security measures. If possible, aisle or exit row seating should be arranged for tall athletes to allow more comfortable leg room. Physically disabled athletes may require special seating or transportation arrangements. Loose fitting, comfortable clothing is recommended. Flight delays, layovers, and lost luggage can cause undue anxiety, and coping strategies are encouraged, including bringing music for personal listening enjoyment, books or magazines to read, and meditation or self-hypnosis [7,9,10,14]. Before boarding flights, it is recommended to avoid ingesting large amounts of caffeine, alcohol, or food.

On board, athletes are likely to be immobile for long periods, which may lead to an increased risk of venous thromboembolism [17,18]. It is advisable to initiate prophylactic measures against venous stasis during long flights, such as walking around the cabin at least once per hour, wearing lower-leg support stockings, and performing isometric exercises of the lower leg while seated. The role for aspirin in the prevention of air travel–related thromboembolism has not been substantiated and may be of limited efficacy [19].

Rapid travel across several time zones is associated with an entity known as jet lag [12–15,20]. The diagnostic criteria for this disorder are outlined in the *International Classification of Sleep Disorders* [21]. Symptoms include daytime fatigue on arrival in the new time zone and trouble sleeping at night, irritability, concentration difficulties, decreased energy and motivation, headaches, decreased appetite, and bowel irregularities [20,21]. This constellation of symptoms is usually worse with eastward travel versus westward travel and depends on the number of time zones crossed [15]. Athletes have been found to be susceptible to the effects of jet lag when traveling to international competition [13].

Inhalant

Albuterol
Triamcinolone
Amonia

Injectable

Dextrose
Diazepam
Diphenhydramine
Epinephrine
Furosemide
Glucagon
Sumatriptan
Triamcinolone
Ketorolac
Lidocaine
Lorazepam
Marcaine
Promethazine

Suppository

Promethazine
Trimethobenzamide

Ophthalmic

Saline Eye Wash
Azelastine
Sulfacetamide
Ciprofloxacin
Homatropine
Tetracaine

Topical

Corticosteroid creams
(high, medium, low potency)
Lidocaine
Mupirocin
Clotrimazole

Oral

Acetaminophen
Acetaminophen/Codeine
Aspirin
Cyclobenzaprine
Prednisone
Diphenhydramine
Enalapril
Hydrocodone/Acetaminophen
Ibuprofen
Loperamide
Lorazepam
Naproxen
Esomeprazole
Nitroglycerin
Prochlorperazine maleate
Promethazine
Trimethoprim/Sulfamethoxazole
Metoprolol
Tramadol
Glucose
Cephalexin
Levofloxacin

Fig. 3. Suggested medications for the medical kit.

The underlying cause of jet lag is thought to be related to a desynchrony of the body's natural circadian rhythm as it attempts to adjust to a new time zone [13,20]. It has been suggested that athletic performance is transiently impaired by the effects of jet lag [11,12,14,22]; however, there is little scientific evidence, specifically randomized controlled trials, supporting this premise [16,23].

Despite the lack of quality scientific evidence, there are certain recommendations for traveling athletes based on expert opinion that may be helpful and should not be harmful to performance. Any adjustments made to alleviate the effects of jet lag should factor in direction of travel, number of time zones crossed, and time of arrival. Traditionally, one day of adjustment is required for each time zone crossed; however, there is great individual variation [10,15,24]. Sleep hygiene should be a focus of intervention, including avoiding sleep deprivation before travel, gradually shifting sleep schedule toward the new schedule based on the time zone of destination, and choosing a flight

Medications

- Personal prescription medications (copies of all prescriptions, including the generic names for medications, and a note from the prescribing physician on letterhead stationary for controlled substances and injectable medications should be carried)
- Antimalarial medications, if applicable
- Antidiarrheal medication (e.g., bismuth subsalicylate, loperamide)
- Antibiotic for self-treatment of moderate to severe diarrhea
- Antihistamine
- Decongestant, alone or in combination with antihistamine
- Antimotion sickness medication
- Acetaminophen, aspirin, ibuprofen, or other medication for pain or fever
- Mild laxative
- Cough suppressant/expectorant
- Throat lozenges
- Antacid
- Antifungal and antibacterial ointments or creams
- 1% hydrocortisone cream
- Epinephrine auto-injector (e.g., EpiPen), especially if history of severe allergic reaction. Also available in smaller-dose package for children.

Other Important Items

- Insect repellent containing DEET (up to 50%)
- Sunscreen (preferably SPF 15 or greater)
- Aloe gel for sunburns
- Digital thermometer
- Oral rehydration solution packets
- Basic first-aid items (adhesive bandages, gauze, ace wrap, antiseptic, tweezers, scissors, cotton-tipped applicators)
- Antibacterial hand wipes or alcohol-based hand sanitizer
- Moleskin for blisters
- Lubricating eye drops (e.g., Natural Tears)
- First Aid Quick Reference card

Other items that may be useful in certain circumstances

- Mild sedative (e.g., zolpidem) or other sleep aid
- Anti-anxiety medication
- High-altitude preventive medication
- Water purification tablets
- Commercial suture/syringe kits (to be used by local health-care provider. These items will also require a letter from the prescribing physician on letterhead stationary)
- Latex condoms
- Address and phone numbers of area hospitals or clinics

Fig. 4. *From* Centers for Disease Control and Prevention. Health information for international travel 2008. Atlanta: US Department of Health and Human Services, Public Health Service, 2007.

schedule that allows for the shortest amount of time possible between destination arrival and going to sleep for a full night of sleep in the new time zone [13,15,23]. Adjustment of personal timepieces to the time zone of destination before boarding or during midflight may help with adjustment. The timing and type of meals has been considered as a way to cope with jet lag, specifically the "feeding hypothesis," which promotes high protein foods for breakfast and

Country: _____
2006 IWF Masters Medical Information Form

Please fill out in English
May be filled out by Lifter, Lifter's representative or Physician
Return with Registration

Name: _____ **Date of Birth:** _____ **Age:**_____years
        Last name   *First Name*   *Month/Day/Year*

Home Address: _____
            Street   City   State/Province   Country

Telephone number: _____ **Date of Last Exam by Physician:**_____

What languages do you speak? :_____

CURRENT MEDICATIONS:
(list with current dosage):
1)   3)   5)
2)   4)   6)

ALLERGIES: _____

PAST SURGERY:
(year & types of all surgeries)
1)   3)   5)
2)   4)   6)

PAST & CURRENT MEDICAL PROBLEMS:
(list year occurred, **circle** if current or past problem) (*example: 1) 1999 High Blood Pressure past* **current**)
1)   past current 3)   past current 5)   past current
2)   past current 4)   past current 6)   past current

Please answer the following questions:
1) **Do you smoke Tobacco?** Yes No *(circle one)*
        if yes: A) How many years have you smoked? _____ years
                  B) How many cigars/cigarettes/pipes do you smoke a day? _____/day

2) **Do you have Diabetes (high blood sugar) ?** Yes No *(circle one)*
        if yes: A) What year were you diagnosed?
                  B) How is it controlled? *(circle all that apply)*
                  Diet   *Oral Medication*   *Sub-cutaneous Insulin*   *Insulin pump*   *Not controlled*

3) **Do you have Heart trouble?** Yes No *(circle one)*
        If yes: A) Have you had a heart attack (myocardial infarction)? Yes No *(circle one)*
                       If yes: Date_____ Did you have surgery? Yes No *(circle one)*

4) **Have you ever had a stroke (cerebral vascular accident)?** Yes No *(circle one)*
        If yes: A) Date of Stroke:_____ Any persisting symptoms?_____

5) **Have you ever dislocated your shoulder or elbow?** Yes No *(circle one)*
        if yes: A) Year(s) that dislocations occurred? _____
                  B) Did you have surgery? Yes No *(circle one)*

IMPORTANT: this questionnaire is confidential and will be used by the IWF Masters medical team in case of injury during the competition. This form will NOT be used to qualify or disqualify a lifter in terms of their health status. All lifters are recommended to see their own personal physician to address their health status prior to engaging in this competition.
Please sign stating the above information is correct to the best of your knowledge.
Name of person filling out this form: _____
Signature of person filling out this form: _____

Fig. 5. Emergency medical form. (*Courtesy of* International Weightlifting Federation, Budapest, Hungary; with permission.)

Athletic Injury Report
International Weightlifting Federation
2006 Masters World Championships

Date:_____ Time:_____ AM/PM Competition/Location:__Bordeaux, FRANCE__

Patient's Name: _____ Sex: _____ D.O.B.:_____
               Last   First

Address: _____
         City   State   Country

Present Rx Medication:_____Allergies:_____

Surgical/ Medical Hx:_____ Date of Onset:_____

Injured Area/ complaint:_____ Acute Chronic Both

Occurred During: Training   Pre-Event/ Warm-up   Travel   Other_____

During Event   Snatch   Clean & Jerk   Attempt 1 2 3

SubjectiveComplaints:_____
_____
_____

Objective Findings:
_____
_____
_____

Assessment/ Diagnosis:_____

Plan/Treatment:_____
_____
_____

Is athlete able to continue competition? Yes No
Is athlete refered for further evaluation? Yes No Where?:_____

Evaluator:_____ Date _____

Fig. 6. Injury report form. (*Courtesy of* International Weightlifting Federation, Budapest, Hungary; with permission.)

high carbohydrate foods for dinner. Theoretically, proteins would provide substrate for arousal neurotransmitters like noradrenaline and dopamine, whereas carbohydrates would promote release of serotonin, a precursor of melatonin, which may help promote sleep [10,14]. There is little scientific evidence to support this theory, and athletes may be better off consuming foods to which they are accustomed and synchronizing their meals with the destination time zone. Athletes should consider avoiding heavy training on arrival and instead participate in one or two light training sessions to ease their transition.

    Pharmacologic therapies have been investigated to alleviate the effects of jet lag. Drugs such as modafinil, amphetamines, and pemoline have been shown to increase levels of alertness and promote mental performance. Their use may be acceptable for noncompeting members of the traveling team, but these drugs should not be used by athletes because they are on the International Olympic Committee and World Anti-Doping Agency list of banned substances [15]. Caffeine is also known to be a stimulant and may help promote alertness on arrival. Its use is not strictly prohibited in athletes, and slow-release caffeine may limit impairment in physical performance associated with jet lag [25]. Benzodiazepines have a hypnotic and somnolent effect that can be helpful in promoting sleep when taken before bedtime or during a long flight. The residual side effects of drowsiness and decreased psychomotor performance, however, are detrimental to athletic performance [10]. Sleep aids such as benzodiazepines, zolpidem, and zaleplon should only be used in traveling athletes who have persistent insomnia and have used them before and know the effects on their body. Their use should always be directed and guided by a sports medicine physician or sports psychiatrist.

Melatonin is a hormone synthesized from serotonin, which is released from the pineal gland and known to have hypnotic and hypothermic effects. Secretion of melatonin occurs primarily at night, is inhibited by bright light, and seems to play a key role in circadian rhythms [10,14,15,24,26,27]. It has been shown to alleviate the subjective feelings of jet lag [24]. There has been conflicting evidence in the literature as to its effect on athletic performance when used for the amelioration of jet lag symptoms [23,25,26,28]. It can have deleterious effects of drowsiness and headaches in some individuals and may hinder performance if not taken in appropriate doses or at the correct time. As with other sleep aids, athletes should only use melatonin during travel to competition if they have used it before and are familiar with its effect on their body [26]. Detailed advice concerning dosing and timing of administration can be found in position statements by the British Olympic Association and the International Federation of Sports Medicine [23,26].

Airline travel for athletic competitions can interfere significantly with an athlete's normal dietary practices. Airlines generally provide limited access to food or drinks while on board, which means that athletes should be prepared by traveling with preferred foods and beverages for consumption during the flight. Food allergies and specialty meal concerns should be addressed with the airline well in advance of travel and confirmed on check-in [29]. Alcohol and caffeinated beverages should be avoided, whereas water, juice, or sports drinks should be consumed liberally to avoid insidious dehydration. Although the low humidity in planes probably does not contribute directly to clinically significant dehydration, it can cause uncomfortable effects including dry eyes and sore, cracked lips. Lip balms and eye drops can be helpful. Those who wear contacts may want to consider wearing glasses instead.

Finally, on arrival at the final destination, team members must be prepared for the occasional difficulties associated with airline travel, including lost luggage and miscommunication with ground transportation. These delays and potential frustrations should be handled with indifference by athletes to avoid added stress and anxiety. Appointing a coach or team manager to handle such issues may allow athletes to concentrate on preparation for competition. It is also a good idea to allow several days for adjustment to a new country and culture before competition.

COMPETITION

Providing medical coverage for athletes at an international competition presents many logistical issues, whether the competition is on home soil or in another country. Issues concerning the medical coverage of an international sporting event and those faced by individual athletes are discussed in the following paragraphs.

It is important to establish the scope of medical care at the event. Preparations, equipment, and providers needed depend on the size, location, and type of competition. Some competitions require comprehensive medical care for athletes, fans, coaches, officials, and staff, whereas others require only responsibility for athletes. Large events with multiple venues such as the Olympic, Paralympic, or World Masters Games will necessitate many volunteers who have varying levels of training. The authors' experience and that of others at these events has shown that most medical encounters have been of low acuity [30–34]. In addition, several studies have demonstrated that nurses and paramedics can perform effectively in triage and stabilization of medical problems in areas with established emergency medical services (EMS) and under the guidance of standardized orders developed by a physician [30,31,33]. Volunteers may be generalized into two groups: medical providers and first responders. Medical providers are those who have license to dispense medications or are trained in advanced cardiac life support (ACLS). These volunteers include physicians, registered nurses, and paramedics, among others. First providers might include ATCs, emergency medical technicians, licensed practical nurses, Red Cross volunteers, or those who have first aid training. It may also be helpful to classify providers based on their ability to perform cardiopulmonary resuscitation or to operate an automatic external defibrillator (AED). A system should be established that determines the medical risk associated with various venues at these large events. Higher-risk events (American football, rugby, downhill skiing, and so forth) warrant higher-level providers, ACLS equipment, and on-site EMS transport. Lower-risk events (bowling, volleyball, billiards, and so forth) may only require a medical provider and an AED on-site [30]. A triage system should also be established that directs medical providers and first responders on how to respond or triage patients based on the acuity of their medical problem. Thompson and colleagues [31] developed an acuity scoring criteria system based on emergency department triage concepts, which seemed to work fairly well at the Winter Olympic Games in Calgary.

The location of the medical team at each venue should be strategically planned to allow easy access by the athletes. Adequate space and a private area need to be made available for discreet examination and treatment. It is also recommended that the medical area have an unrestricted view of the competitors and direct access to the competition area. This view allows medical staff to see injuries when they occur and to be aware of the mechanism of injury. It also provides for quick access to injured, nonambulatory athletes who may need transported to the medical area. If placement of the medical team is unrealistic due to the nature of the sport or location (eg, triathlon, marathons, and so forth), some members of the medical team should be placed at key locations of the competition to render emergent care and then assist in transfer to the main medical area.

Medical emergencies may not be common at sporting events, but being prepared for their occurrence is vital. The ideal time to consider how an emergency should best be handled is before an emergency occurs. This planning requires communication with the host country to determine what system of emergency medical care is in place. Sporting events held in rural areas may not have EMS or a hospital within close proximity, which requires pre-event planning to have some type of emergency transport available in case of catastrophic injuries. Disaster planning should include an evacuation plan from each venue for natural disasters or terrorist attacks [8,32,35,36]. If feasible, these disaster plans should be coordinated with existing community plans [31]. AEDs should also be available at venues or within a 3-minute response time. Large venues may require multiple AEDs. Motyka and colleagues [37] developed a simple process for determining the number of AEDs needed to provide early defibrillation by first responders in areas in which EMS may not be available or delayed. Events with established EMS and local hospitals should be contacted well in advance to help coordinate appropriate emergency care. In addition, response to emergencies may depend on the type of provider present. Franc-Law [30] developed medical control guidelines for the 2005 World Masters Games, which gave simple, concise guidelines to medical volunteers for responding to various emergent injuries or illnesses such as cardiac arrest, anaphylaxis, and head injuries. The medical control guidelines were essentially standardized orders approved by the chief medical officer and medical committee that gave registered nurses and paramedics the ability to dispense medications and activate EMS without a physician being on-site. First responders could also follow guidelines appropriate to their level of training.

All medical volunteers should be provided with a handbook that outlines important information including standardized orders, how to contact EMS, a list of specialty providers in the area for referral, and directions for documentation of all medical encounters. Documentation of medical encounters is essential to track the use of medical services and to guide future medical coverage planning. Some type of injury or illness report form should be created to document all medical encounters. The injury report form that the authors have used for documenting medical encounters during international competitions in weightlifting (see Fig. 6) can be modified for any sport or event. In addition, the emergency medical forms described earlier can be critical when caring for international athletes whose medical histories may be difficult to obtain due to language barriers or catastrophic injury (see Fig. 5).

Caring for international athletes presents unique challenges because of culture and language differences. The language barrier can be merely inconvenient during assessment of nonemergent medical problems but critically important during emergencies. Before competition, interpretive services should be established and protocols put in place for their use. All medical team members should know how to contact an interpreter and, ideally, interpreters for the major languages spoken at the event should be on-site or at least within 5 minutes of the venue. In the United States and Canada, a "language line" can be used for a fee to provide interpretive services over the phone for virtually any language.

Providing medical services for a group of traveling athletes requires being prepared with a variety of medical supplies and medications. Contents of a traveling medical kit, including medications, were discussed earlier (see Fig. 4) and may need to be adjusted depending on the athletes' needs. Occasionally, on arrival in the destination country, athletes may need certain medicines or supplies that are not contained in the medical kit. Knowing how the host country's medical system functions, including pharmacy regulations, may prove very useful. Often, medications or supplies that require a prescription to purchase in the home country can be purchased as an over-the-counter item without a prescription from a local pharmacy.

Adjustment to a different country and culture, along with issues of diet, hydration, rest, and acclimatization, is faced by athletes during an international event. The cultural experience is an important part of the athletic event but should not overshadow the competition preparation. Athletes should make smart decisions regarding how much sightseeing or walking is done before competing. Excessive standing or walking during opening ceremonies or spectating at other venues can potentially lead to poor performances on the day of competition. Adequate rest should be scheduled into the daily routine, including naps if necessary.

Precautions taken before enjoying local cuisine will help prevent diarrheal illness, which can lead to dehydration and fatigue. Traveler's diarrhea is common in developing countries and can be avoided by frequent hand washing, drinking bottled or purified water, adequate cooking of food, and not eating unwashed fruits or vegetables. If contracted, antibiotics in the fluoroquinolone class are first-line treatment because most traveler's diarrhea is caused by bacteria [5,9]. Care should be taken in strength athletes who are on fluoroquinolones because of the risk of tendon rupture [38]. Adequate oral fluid resuscitation should also be emphasized, in the form of bottled water or sports drinks, to prevent dehydration.

POST COMPETITION

After the athletic competition and before travel home, the same precautions and advice discussed for travel to the event should be reviewed with the medical team, athletes, and staff. Any athletes who suffered illness or injury should be monitored closely on the trip home, and accommodations for their care at home arranged ahead of time. The head physician or medical director should assemble a report of all medical encounters, including type of injury or illness, treatments, and need for EMS or ambulance transport. This report should also review the medical protocols and guidelines used during the event and whether any changes should be made in the future. This report can be presented to the event organizer or local organizing committee to summarize all medical care provided at the event. Completing this step helps to justify why your services were needed, engenders goodwill, and allows for better preparation by the event organizer for subsequent competitions.

On arrival in the home country, a debriefing session should be organized by the head physician to review important issues raised by competition coverage and changes that might need to be made for the future medical care of athletes during international competitions [7]. Individual athletes may benefit from reviewing their international athletic experience and documenting the strategies that worked well for them in combating travel fatigue and optimizing their athletic performance.

References

[1] Mast E, Goodman R. Prevention of infectious disease transmission in sports. Sports Med 1997;24(1):1–7.

[2] Ehresmann K, Hedberg C, Grimm M, et al. An outbreak of measles at an international sporting event with airborne transmission in a domed stadium. J Infect Dis 1995;171:679–83.

[3] Goodman R, Thacker S, Solomon S, et al. Infectious diseases in competitive sports. JAMA 1994;271(11):862–7.

[4] Turbeville S, Cowan L, Greenfield R. Infectious disease outbreaks in competitive sports: a review of the literature. Am J Sports Med 2006;34(11):1860–5.

[5] CDC. Recommendations for travelers: being prepared in case disaster strikes. Available at: http://www.cdc.gov/travel/other/2006/disasterprep.htm. Accessed October 16, 2006.

[6] Shaw M, Leggat P. Traveling to Australia for the Sydney 2000 Olympic and Paralympic games. J Travel Med 2000;7:200–4.

[7] Milne C, Shaw M, Steinweg J. Medical issues relating to the Sydney Olympic Games. Sports Med 1999;28(4):287–98.

[8] Herring S, Bergfeld J, Boyd J, et al. Sideline preparedness for the team physician: a consensus statement. Med Sci Sports Exerc 2001;33(5):846–9.

[9] Young M, Fricker P, Maughan R, et al. The traveling athlete: issues relating to the Commonwealth Games, Malaysia, 1998. Br J Sports Med 1998;32:77–81.

[10] Waterhouse J, Reilly T, Edwards B. The stress of travel. J Sports Sci 2004;22:946–66.

[11] Hill D, Hill C, Fields K, et al. Effects of jet lag on factors related to sport performance. Can J Appl Physiol 1993;18(1):91–103.

[12] Manfredini R, Manfredini F, Fersini C, et al. Circadian rhythms, athletic performance, and jet lag. Br J Sports Med 1998;32:101–6.

[13] Waterhouse J, Edwards B, Nevill A, et al. Identifying some determinants of "jet lag" and its symptoms: a study of athletes and other travelers. Br J Sports Med 2002;36:54–60.

[14] Reilly T, Atkinson G, Waterhouse J. Travel fatigue and jet-lag. J Sports Sci 1997;15:365–9.

[15] Reilly T, Waterhouse J. Jet lag and air travel: implications for performance. Clin Sports Med 2005;24:367–80.

[16] Youngstedt S, O'Connor P. The influence of air travel on athletic performance. Sports Med 1999;28(3):197–207.

[17] Ansari M, Cheung B, Qing Huang J, et al. Traveler's thrombosis: a systemic review. J Travel Med 2005;12(3):142–54.

[18] Hughes R, Hopkins R, Hill S, et al. Frequency of venous thromboembolism in low to moderate risk long distance air travelers: the New Zealand Air Traveller's Thrombosis (NZATT) study. Lancet 2003;362(9401):2039–44.

[19] Hovens M, Snoep J, Tamsma J, et al. Aspirin in the prevention and treatment of venous thromboembolism. J Thromb Haemost 2006;4(7):1470–5.

[20] Waterhouse J, Reilly T, Atkinson G. Jet lag. Lancet 1997;350(9091):1611–6.

[21] Thorpy J. International classification of sleep disorders, revised: diagnostic and coding manual. Westchester (IL): American Academy of Sleep Medicine; 2001.

[22] Drust B, Waterhouse J, Atkinson G. Circadian rhythms in sports performance: an update. Chronobiol Int 2005;22(1):21–44.

[23] O'Connor P, Youngstedt S, Buxton O, et-al. Air travel and performance in sports. Position statement: the International Federation of Sports Medicine 2004. Available at: http://www.fims.org. Accessed October 16, 2006.

[24] Atkinson G, Drust B, Reilly R, et al. The relevance of melatonin to sports medicine and science. Sports Med 2003;33(11):809–31.

[25] Lagarde D, Chappuis B, Billaud P. Evaluation of pharmacological aids on physical performance after a transmeridian flight. Med Sci Sports Exerc 2001;33(4):628–34.

[26] Waterhouse J, Reilly T, Atkinson G. Melatonin and jet lag. Br J Sports Med 1998;32:98–100.

[27] Herxheimer A, Petrie K. Melatonin for the prevention and treatment of jet lag. In: The Cochrane library. Oxford (UK): Update Software; 2006.

[28] Atkinson G, Buckley P, Edwards B, et al. Are there hangover-effects on physical performance when melatonin is ingested by athletes before nocturnal sleep? Int J Sports Med 2001;22:232–4.

[29] Leggat P, Nowak M. Dietary advice for airline travel. J Travel Med 1997;4:14–6.

[30] Franc-Law J. A community-based model for medical management of a large scale sporting event. Clin J Sport Med 2006;16:406–11.

[31] Thompson J, Savoia G, Powell G, et al. Level of medical care required for mass gatherings: the XV Winter Olympic games in Calgary, Canada. Ann Emerg Med 1991;20:385–90.

[32] Wetterhall S, Coulombier D, Herndon J, et al. Medical care delivery at the 1996 Olympic Games. JAMA 1998;279:1463–8.

[33] McDonald C, Koenigsberg M, Ward S. Medical control of mass gatherings: can paramedics perform without physicians on-site? Prehospital Disaster Med 1993;8(4):327–31.

[34] Weiss B, Mascola L, Fannin S. Public health at the 1984 Summer Olympics: the Los Angeles county experience. Am J Public Health 1988;78:686–8.

[35] Hadjichristodoulou C, Mouchtouri V, Soteriades E, et al. Mass gathering preparedness: the experience of the Athens 2004 Olympic and Paralympic games. J Environ Health 2005;67(9):52–7.

[36] Jorm L, Visotina M. Keeping the dream alive and healthy: public health preparations for the Sydney 2000 Olympic and Paralympic Games. NSW Public Health Bull 2000;11(8):137–57.

[37] Motyka T, Winslow J, Newton K, et al. Method for determining automatic external defibrillator need at mass gatherings. Resuscitation 2005;65:309–14.

[38] Van Der Linder P, Sturkenboom M, Herings R, et al. Fluoroquinolone and risk of Achilles tendon disorders: case control study. Br J Med 2002;324(7349):1304–11.

Clin Sports Med 26 (2007) 505–508

CLINICS IN SPORTS MEDICINE

ELSEVIER
SAUNDERS

INDEX

Note: Page numbers of article titles are in **boldface** type.

0278-5919/07/$ – see front matter
doi:10.1016/S0278-5919(07)00068-3

Moving?

Make sure your subscription moves with you!

To notify us of your new address, find your **Clinics Account Number** (located on your mailing label above your name), and contact customer service at:

E-mail: elspcs@elsevier.com

800-654-2452 (subscribers in the U.S. & Canada)
407-345-4000 (subscribers outside of the U.S. & Canada)

Fax number: 407-363-9661

Elsevier Periodicals Customer Service
6277 Sea Harbor Drive
Orlando, FL 32887-4800

*To ensure uninterrupted delivery of your subscription, please notify us at least 4 weeks in advance of move.